The 3D Diet

Dynamic Dining Design
(Or The Sleep Apnea Diet)

NOT a Diet
A Plan for Life

Lose Weight, Get Healthy
Never Look Back

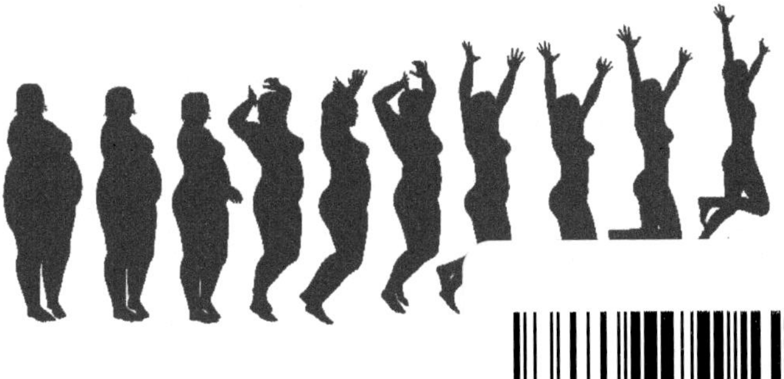

AF887742

By

Victoria Rosenthal

The 3D Diet challenges the established principles of the diet industry and the (*so-called*) medical experts, in a book for **every single person** who has tried every diet there is and ***still failed*** **to lose weight and keep it off.**

This book delivers the straight skinny about weight and how to lose it – ***facts that no one else will tell you!***

The 3D Diet shows you how to:

- identify the medical problems that are keeping you from losing weight;
- how to get the most effective treatment for those medical issues;
- and that you ***really CAN*** eat all you want **and still lose weight!**

Whether you need to lose 5 pounds, 100 pounds or more, **The 3D Diet** will help you **lose the weight** and **keep it off** ***forever!*** You can finally ***BE*** **the brand new beautiful you,** ***you were always meant to be!***

Wicked Read Productions LLC

Publisher

www.WickedReadProductions.com

First published in paperback 2017

ISBN: 0-9988411-9-6
ISBN-13: 978-0-9988411-9-9

Library of Congress Control Number/LCCN: 2017904997
Wicked Read Productions, LLC, St Petersburg, FL

Author: Victoria Rosenthal
Illustrations: Miranda Fegan

Wicked Read Productions, LLC, Publisher
Carson City, NV

Dedication

This book is for everyone who, like me,
struggles with their weight;
with no help whatsoever from
the medical industry, the pharmaceutical industry,
the food industry, the insurance industry, or the
government. Shame on all of them!

And to my wonderful husband, Bruce,
who has been there from size 5
to size 26 and every size in between,
who just simply loves me every single day.

CONTENTS

FOREWORD

This book is for every single person who has ever tried a diet and failed, OR who gained back the weight they lost **plus** a few extra pounds. It is especially for those who have tried diet after diet after diet and failed, gaining back a few pounds more than they lost each and every time.

I am not a medical professional (and I don't play one on TV), I'm not a nutritionist and I'm not a fitness guru. Or, perhaps it is more accurate to say that I have never formally trained in or worked professionally in any of these capacities. But through years of dealing with my own weight problems, spending hundreds of thousands of hours on research, a great deal of trial and error, and a few happy accidents, I have actually ***become*** all of these things and more.

I am just like you – someone who has spent most of my life battling a weight problem. I have clothes in my closet ranging from size 5 (when I weighed 118) to a size 5 XL (when I weighed 284, which I will hopefully never weigh again). All of these clothes remain in my closet because I have cycled through numerous sizes too many times to count as my weight has see-sawed up and down through the years. I can't afford to keep buying a new wardrobe every time my weight changes.

Revolutionary information contained in this book will help you make your own body repair and reboot the systems that are ***supposed*** to naturally regulate your weight so they work properly. Then the thin, healthy person locked inside you will finally emerge.

There is a great deal of information in this book that the mainstream medical community and/or the FDA either won't tell you at all, OR won't tell you in a way that is useful or meaningful. In fact, some of the information in this book is information that the medical community and/or the FDA has specifically tried to understate as insignificant or withhold and conceal. The revelations in this book will leave you gasping, and wondering why no one ever told you this before.

While this book does contain information and advice for people with some very specific types of health and weight management issues, it also contains information that is universally applicable to everyone who has an ongoing weight problem whether you need to lose 5 pounds, 50 pounds, 150 pounds or even more.

If this book helps even one person lose the weight they need to lose and keep it off, then the time and effort that went into writing it was absolutely worthwhile.

FAIRY TALES DOCTORS TELL US
(Or - Liar, Liar, Pants On Fire)

I have known for most of my life that I was not "normal" at least as far as my weight was concerned. I began to suspect something was out of whack with my metabolism (although I didn't know this word at the time) as early as age 7. What I did know was that other girls ate more than I did and were thinner than me.

By the time I was a teenager I was certain something was wrong, but no doctor would agree with me. By age 22 I was angry, and see-saw weight gains and losses were driving me crazy. By age 30 I was searching for answers with a tenacity that was rivaled only by *The Little Engine that Could.* By age 40 my weight stopped seeing and only sawed as my waist line expanded frighteningly out of control, and still no doctor could or would tell me anything that actually helped.

THE BIG LIE!

Calories IN ***(Food Eaten)***

MINUS **Calories BURNED** ***(Exercise)***

Equals ***YOUR WEIGHT***

How many times have you heard this? I have actually sat in doctors' offices – doctors to whom I was paying good money to help me solve my weight problems – and had the (usually obnoxiously thin, robustly healthy) physician give me a knowing smirk and a sad little shake of the head over my obvious (to them) delusional state as they utter this trite lie. It makes me want to scream (or more satisfyingly, punch out their lights). I even had doctors talk to me seriously about lap bands and gastric by-pass surgery.

Convincing these medical morons that your weight is **NOT** about what goes in your mouth is frequently a losing battle. If this happens to you (and it will), you might as well forfeit your "initial visit" fee, leave, and go to the next doctor on your list.

If you are like me, you **KNOW** this tired old cliché isn't true. It can't be. Lots of people eat far more than I do, get even less exercise and ***STILL*** weigh far less.

My own mother ate like a horse and never gained an ounce. She was 5'7" and never weighed more than a fairly steady 124 pounds no matter what she ate (until she was post-menopausal). This is a woman who, after a hearty breakfast, a lavish lunch and a marathon dinner (meals punctuated throughout the day with bunches of grapes, slices of watermelon and a slice or three of key lime pie), would then for a late night snack polish off an entire family sized box of Mrs. Paul's fried scallops or half a pan of cornbread and two or three glasses of milk (whole milk mind you, not that nasty skim or reduced fat stuff I choked down) and she never gained an ounce! It was maddening!

Don't get me wrong, I loved my mother – she was my best friend. But it was hard watching her eat (especially when I was a teenager and my mother was in her late forties); ***KNOWING*** that if I ate in a week what she ate in one day I would blow up to the size of the Goodyear blimp.

We ALL know women (or men) like this. Women (or men) with *SEEMINGLY* **"MAGIC" genes**. I have had friends and acquaintances and co-workers and frienemies who could stuff their faces from morning to night with hamburgers and fries and ice cream and whatever else their little hearts (or stomachs) desired. Occasionally these women with their God given ***magic genes*** get concerned about the pesky 5 pounds they need to drop after the "holidays" wherein they consumed everything but the table legs at Thanksgiving dinner, managed to daintily wolf down enough to feed Santa and all of this elves during Christmas, and polished off New Year's by chucking down enough hors d' oeuvres, dinner, and champagne to satisfy half of the crowd in Time Square.

Where the hell are my magic genes? I want to know! I need answers! Why is it that if I so much as ***LOOK*** at a piece of pizza, 5 pounds maliciously appear on my hips?!!

And now this smug, arrogant doctor has the temerity to smirk at me over his desk and tell me if I just eat less my problems will resolve themselves???

Maybe the old calories in, calories out thing is true for normal people, but it sure isn't true for me.

The whole point of this book is to help others like me. To share the answers I have discovered, and help you understand some of the things no one else will tell you that are causing you to gain weight, OR, more to the point, making it IMPOSSIBLE for you to lose weight.

AN UNDECLARED EPIDEMIC OF EPIC PROPORTION

(Double Entendre Intended)

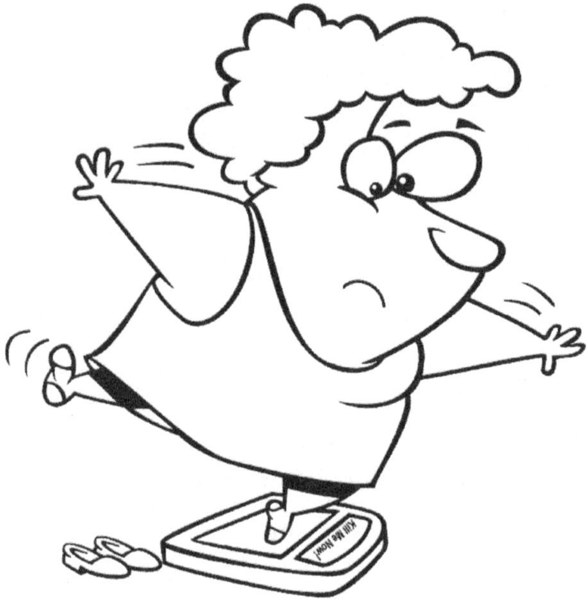

As I write this book, according to the U.S. Centers for Disease Control National Center for Health Statistics 2013-2014 statistics over 70% percent of the population of the United States is overweight; over 37% of the population is classified as medically obese. Sadly more than 17% percent of the population is diagnosed as morbidly obese. The global statistics are even more frightening. According to the World Health Organization's 2014 statistics over 1.9 Billion adults are overweight or obese and more than 65% of the world's population lives in countries where **being overweight KILLS** many times the number of people who die of starvation.

How can this be true? Especially in the United States where we have the best medical care in the world . . . or so they tell us.

In the United States alone the Diet Industry is a $65+ Billion per year industry; and that figure represents ***ONLY*** what is spent on weight loss products, foods, and services.

But the $65+ Billion is really only the tip of the iceberg. It is impossible to determine exactly how much is spent each year on medical services, prescription medications and surgeries due to obesity because the reason for medical intervention is usually reported as something *OTHER* than obesity, or is reported as a condition that is a result of obesity, rather than reporting the reason as obesity itself.

As with many other problems plaguing our society today, there are a number of big business interests that shamelessly exploit and capitalize on various things that contribute to the obesity problem. As you read further, you will see that many of the problems causing obesity (at least in the U.S.) are primarily due to corporate greed hand in hand with a government and an FDA that respond more readily to the money these corporations pour into government coffers than any real thought or concern for the needs of individual citizens, especially those of us who are struggling with weight problems.

Many of the issues fall into the "follow the money" category, where numerous interested parties are conspiring to insure the continued financial success of their product, company, industry or government agency at our expense.

So many of the health problems primarily caused by obesity are so vehemently and systematically disassociated with obesity by the medical community, that the vehement disassociation itself is suspicious.

Type 2 Diabetes and Insulin Resistance were once relatively rare in this country. Today both are epidemic and both are a direct result of the obesity problem. According to a study published in the September 2000 issue of Diabetes Care (Table 3, Pg 1280), between 1990 and 1998 alone there was a 70% increase in Type 2 Diabetes in adults between 30 and 39; there was a 40% increase in adults between 40 and 49.

Type 2 Diabetes almost always develops in adulthood. It is generally caused by too much insulin not being properly utilized due to insulin resistance.

Insulin Resistance most often develops due to consumption of high glucose carbohydrates, and is frequently the combined result of obesity and a diet high in pasta, bread, bagels, fruit juice, candy, soda, pastries, etc.

The high blood sugar caused by Type 2 Diabetes (OR by a PRE-Type 2 Diabetic condition) causes your body to rapidly store excess fat, generates extreme hunger, and will absolutely, without question insure that you gain weight with the speed of light. If you are "Hyper-sugar" or have Type 2 Diabetes and have **NOT** yet been diagnosed, it is urgent that you see a doctor and get on proper medication immediately.

Another medical problem hardly ever heard of 50 years ago, that is increasing at alarming rates, is High Cholesterol. Scientists have finally acknowledged that High Cholesterol is ***NOT*** the result of eating foods that contain cholesterol (such as eggs). Having High Cholesterol indicates that your body ***is not processing food properly***, and you will have High

Cholesterol, regardless of what you eat, until the underlying problem is corrected.

Interestingly, (or disturbingly) the level of cholesterol that is ***CONSIDERED*** to be medically "high" by the health care industry has ***CONTINUOUSLY*** been adjusted **downward** as more and more expensive medications designed to lower cholesterol (such as statins) have come on the market.

The medical community almost ***NEVER*** tells anyone that it is possible to correct High Cholesterol **without** the use of statins. I'll bet your doctor has **never** told you that Hypothyroidism is one of the leading causes, and may very well be the #1 leading cause, of High Cholesterol, even though it is well documented by respected organizations from the Mayo Clinic on down that High Cholesterol is a **SYMPTOM** of Hypothyroidism. In fact, the American Association of Clinical Endocrinologists guidelines require screening for Hypothyroidism when diagnosing a patient with High Cholesterol, but studies have shown that this protocol is followed only approximately 50% of the time. If you are one of the tens of millions of people who have a **Thyroid Disorder** that is **UNDIAGNOSED**, it is highly likely the undiagnosed Thyroid Disorder is the root cause of your High Cholesterol.

The most important thing is that being overweight does **NOT** necessarily mean you overeat. ***The assertion that* "everyone who is overweight overeats" *is the biggest, most insidious lie we have been told.*** And I am sure you have heard it over and over ad nauseam for decades.

All my life (and probably for years before I was born) smug medical "experts" have told overweight people that we eat too much and exercise too little. They have shouted this from the mountain tops and made us feel ashamed, as if it is our own fault that our body doesn't work correctly and medical science has failed us.

There is no reason to be ashamed! The government and the FDA, in collusion with the very wealthy food industry, have created this situation. The medical community has supported these institutions and has chosen to keep us fat rather than correctly diagnosing our medical problems and helping us.

It's time to fight back. You **CAN** lose weight. All you need is the right information, which you will find in this book.

Losing weight, or trying to lose weight, is one of the world's most frustrating, thankless battles. After all, we are fighting 20 Million years of evolution, outright lies and deception on the part of the government and the medical community, as well as 21st Century corporate and government greed. However it is critical that you lose weight in order to restore your health. Being overweight or obese isn't just an "ok, so I'm overweight" kind of problem. It is a serious physical condition that is extremely detrimental to your lifelong health and wellbeing.

SYMPTOMS OF CHRONIC OBESITY
(Include, but are not limited to)

- Thyroid disorders (yes, obesity can actually ***cause*** thyroid disorders)
- Insulin resistance
- Sugar Addiction

- Always hot or cold when others are comfortable
- Inability to lose weight eating diet on which others are slim
- Eating for comfort
- Over eating
- Extreme hunger for no good reason
- Lack of Serotonin and Melatonin
- Difficulty Breathing
- Shortness of Breath
- Difficulty Walking or Running
- Increased Sweating
- Pain in Knee and Ankle Joints
- Back Pain
- Acne
- Acid Reflux/GERDS Syndrome
- High Blood Pressure
- Sleep Apnea
- Lack of Sex Drive
- Heart Attack
- Stroke
- Increased Risk of Mortality
- Early Death

- Psychological Damage
    - Low Self-Esteem
    - Social Anxiety
    - Poor body Image
    - Depression

SERIOUS HEALTH CONDITIONS CAUSED BY OBESITY

(Include, but are not limited to)

- Thyroid Disorders
- Metabolic Syndrome
- Impaired Adrenal Function
- Sleep Apnea
- Insomnia
- Restless Leg Syndrome
- Hyper Sugar
- Hypoglycemia
- Inability of body to utilize insulin correctly
- Diabetes Type 2
- Fibromyalgia
- Joint Pain
- Osteoarthritis

- Back Injury
- Sexual Dysfunction
- Impaired Liver Function
- Fatty Liver
- Diverticulitis
- Gallstones
- High Cholesterol
- Hardening of the Arteries
- Cardiac Disease
- Certain Types of Cancer
- Death

All of these problems are correctable, ***IF*** you lose weight before something irreversible occurs, like heart attack, stroke, or death.

This book contains the information no one has ever told you that will help you lose the weight permanently. You will finally be able to slim down to the weight you are supposed to be; be able to eat like a normal person; and be the healthy, beautiful you, you are meant to be.

BUT SHE HAS A GREAT PERSONALITY . . .

It has been scientifically, statistically proven that most people believe individuals who are overweight are unsightly, slovenly and apathetic about their appearance. This leads to substantial discrimination against those of us struggling with weight problems. Even individuals who are overweight *themselves* have been shown to discriminate against other overweight individuals!

The fact of the matter is that most people who are overweight, especially those who have chronic weight problems, care very much about their body, their appearance, and their health. However many of them are discouraged to the point of despair by years of chronic diet failure and the constant humiliation they face from medical professionals, co-workers, friends and family who insist on believing that being overweight ipso facto means you overeat (or even worse, you are secretly bingeing). Most unenlightened normal weight people, including doctors who should know better, flatly **REFUSE** to believe that there are or could be undiagnosed, underlying medical issues causing our weight problems.

I've been overweight most of my life, punctuated by a few brief, but memorable, periods of thinness that occurred at times I was able to momentarily punish my body severely enough to achieve a glorious state of thin.

After I passed my 40th birthday and my weight began to spiral out of control from "plump" to seriously obese, my own mother began to frequently pull me aside and talk to me in a hushed, sorrowful voice about my eating habits. She kept warning me of the dangers to my health and chastising me for (obviously) secretly binge eating when I was alone. She made a point of telling me that such behavior wasn't ***really*** a secret since everyone could clearly see the results! Sheesh! As if I hadn't spent my entire life on a diet, or I didn't know I was fat!

It is a sad commentary on the medical profession that many doctors are either too entrenched in the same attitudes as my mother, too cowed by rules in their contract with your medical insurance company, or are simply too lazy to do the difficult work necessary to diagnose elusive metabolism conditions or other difficult to diagnose health problems that could be negatively affecting your body's ability to properly regulate your weight. Worse, doctors are being ***PAID*** by your medical insurance company to ignore critical disorders affecting your health, and the Obamacare legislation will only further exacerbate this problem over the long term.

It has become so commonplace for doctors to refuse to accept new patients ***because*** the patient is overweight; the August 2011 issue of Glamour Magazine ran a reader poll asking if this practice was fair on the part of the doctors! A shocking 47% of readers responded that ***YES, this practice is fair and ethical!!*** One doctor interviewed for the article ***freely admitted in print*** that she turned away patients who are overweight because such patients require more procedures and tests and this factor makes it more likely the Insurance Companies would expel the doctor from their plans!!!

Even more recently, a 2013 study done by Johns Hopkins University found that doctors treated normal weight patients more kindly and empathetically than they treated obese patients. The results showed that most doctors maintain an emotional distance and don't engage in rapport building with obese patients.

For all of these reasons and more, it is crucial for you to insure that any and all health problems that could be inhibiting your ability to lose weight are diagnosed and properly treated. No diet will ever be successful ***REGARDLESS*** of what you eat or do not eat if you have undiagnosed health problems that prevent weight loss. A large percentage of this book is devoted to revealing the health issues no one may ever tell you could be affecting your ability to lose weight, and many of these are types of medical issues which frequently go undiagnosed and may never even be discussed with you or considered by your doctor(s).

What you don't know **CAN** hurt you – and in this case complications or ancillary conditions (such as Type 2 Diabetes) caused by untreated obesity or undiagnosed disorders causing obesity can be fatal.

Achieving proper diagnosis and treatment of your health issues is not always easy. You must first find the right doctor or combination of doctors. Hopefully the information in this book will give you some clue of the direction you should go, and what type of doctor(s) you should consult. Regardless of anything else you may suspect is wrong, you should at least consider seeing a doctor who specializes in obesity and weight loss. However, despite the numerous health problems associated with weight issues, more and more medical insurance policies do **not** cover weight loss specialists.

Be cautious and meticulous if you are choosing a weight loss specialist. Be certain you have thoroughly investigated their credentials, their success record, and if possible that you have talked to some of their patients who are successfully losing weight.

Be leery of doctors who sell their own proprietary blends of vitamins or weight loss supplements, or who sell from their office any brand of weight loss products that cannot be purchased publically. In many instances these types of sales provide a significant revenue stream for the physician and the good doctor cares more about selling you what may be placebos than they care about your actual weight loss or health problems.

Once you have decided on a doctor or weight loss professional you believe can help you, you still need to arm yourself with the knowledge to insure that your issues are taken seriously from the beginning. Since most medical professionals, including weight loss specialists, are strongly biased towards believing that anyone who is overweight is overeating, you don't want to waste precious months and dollars convincing the doctor that overeating is **NOT** the root cause of your weight problem.

Let me suggest that **BEFORE** you go to the first visit with any doctor you should spend a month keeping a detailed food journal. In fact, why wait – start today! This way you will be armed and dangerous when you go to that first visit. Be sure you include every morsel that has passed your lips, including beverages and snacks; see the sample Food Journal further on in this book. To save time and protect against doctors who don't want to believe you, it is a good idea to have your spouse, significant other, roommate or close friend who is frequently with you sign a letter stating that they certify what you have logged in your Journal is the unvarnished truth. It is shocking how many medical professionals accuse overweight people of lying about what they eat.

DIET, DIET, WHO'S GOT THE DIET?

Not surprisingly, with a diet industry that exceeds $65+ Billion annually in the United States alone, the number of diets competing for your diet dollars is staggering. Even a partial list of some of the best known diets ranges from the tried and true (effective for many), such as Weight Watchers or Richard Simmons (who, according to his website, has been responsible for over 3 million pounds lost) – to the logical (diets effective for some people) such as Atkins or Pritkin – to the sublime, such as the Apple Cider Vinegar Diet or the Cabbage Soup Diet (which I personally attest works for the short term, at least until you start eating again) – to the ridiculous, such as the Drinking Man's Diet or the Fast Food Diet (really?).

Just offhand, listing the diets I can remember in three minutes or less, I'll bet the list will include at least half a dozen diets you have tried:

- Weight Watchers – *Diet based on a logical point system for food. In recent years, Weight Watchers also sells food and other diet products.*

- Richard Simmons – *Deal a Meal, Farewell to Fat System and Food Mover Program. These are all based on a reasonable combination of nutritious foods combined with exercise which is both silly and fun.*

- Jenny Craig – *a diet based on buying their food products and joining their gym.*

- The Zone Diet – *a diet 100% based on selling their food products which are conveniently delivered to your door.*
- The South Beach Diet – *Which either requires a commitment to your entire life revolving around cooking* OR *purchasing frozen food products that taste like cardboard.*
- The Atkins Diet
- The Pritkin Diet
- The Apple Cider Vinegar Diet
- The TLC Diet
- Nutri Systems Diet
- The Cabbage Soup Diet
- The Subway Sandwich Diet
- The Carbohydrate Lovers Diet
- The Instinct Diet
- Hollywood Cookie Diet
- Slim Fast
- Medifast
- The Baby Food Diet *(Come on)*
- The Caveman Diet
- The Drinking Man's Diet *(many of us wish this worked)*
- Eat Right for Your Type *(which some people swear by)*
- Eat What You Love Diet *(I wish)*

- The Fast Food Diet
- The Grapefruit Diet
- The Hallelujah Diet
- The Kind Diet *(what?)*
- The Mayo Clinic Diet *(well OK, I once lost a few pounds on this one)*

Did I miss your favorite? There are so many of them it boggles the mind and each one of them has worked for at least one person. I mean, not to malign Subway, but has anyone other than Jared Fogle ever lost weight eating a diet of Subway Sandwiches?

Some of these diets have worked for some people, like the Zone Diet, Jenny Craig, and others. In fact these companies generally run commercials or print ads that show at least four or five people who have lost 40 or 50 pounds or more. ***However*** be sure you catch the disclaimer in microscopic print in the corner, warning you something along the lines of:

"Not Average Results. Everyone loses weight at their own rate."

Some of these diets have worked for thousands of people, like Weight Watchers, Richard Simmons, the Pritkin, the Atkins, etc.

The best diets are based on reasonable nutritional guidelines for the "average" person, some sort of provision for mild exercise, and allow for a little treat every now and again to keep the dieter from giving up completely or committing suicide.

Don't get me wrong – I am not in any way maligning diets that have worked for others. But let's face it, you wouldn't be reading this book (and I wouldn't be writing it) if any of these diets had resulted in positive long term weight loss for us.

When I was 22 a doctor in New York (whose name I no longer recall) gave me a diet he recommended – 600 calories a day based on eating high protein and low carbohydrates. What can you eat for 600 calories a day you might ask? You'd be amazed. I lived on this diet for nearly a decade, and (for at least some of those years) it was the best decade of my life from a weight perspective. It was during this period that I was actually a size 5 for a couple of years. I still have the cut-off jean short shorts that I wore at my very skinniest. My husband frequently suggests I throw them away as they are threadbare, and at the zenith of my weight the ***waist*** of these shorts wouldn't have even closed around one of my thighs. He simply cannot understand that those shorts are a trophy – they once fit me, I looked fabulous in them, AND I have the photographic evidence to prove it!

Of course living on a 600 calorie a day diet is not reasonable, viable, or even advisable for most people and eventually even a diet this extreme didn't work for me anymore.

You will find this book littered with antidotal stories from my own experiences. My experiences eventually lead to finding some answers and to writing this book. Although I know my quest for information is far from over, I believe that most of the readers who purchase this book will identify with many of the things that happened to me in my lifelong struggle to understand why I was gaining weight regardless of what I ate (or more to the point, didn't eat) and irrespective of everything I did to reverse this trend.

The answers I have found so far, I discovered in spite of the obstacles, roadblocks, and outright hostility I have experienced from the medical community who failed to help me even while greedily taking money from me for decades. I truly hope sharing this information will help you and everyone else reading this book.

MY LIFE IN POUNDS
(NO PHOTOS PLEASE!)

When I was five years old some pediatrician told my mother I was undersized for my age and needed to eat more. I wish I knew who he was – I'd sue him for malpractice, although it probably isn't his fault that my metabolism sucks and has plagued me for the last 50+ years.

By age seven I was a chubby little girl (who definitely was no longer undersized for my age); my classmates teased me mercilessly about my weight, and "Fatso" was my nickname for at least a few months. Fortunately, my family moved several times during my school years, and that was one nickname I gladly left behind.

By age twelve, I had come to the realization that if I ate the same things other girls my age ate, I would be fat. So I gave up sweets and junk food and ate the smallest meals my mother would let me get away with. I grew a little taller, slimmed down a bit and looked reasonably decent for my age. But by that time the damage was already done, I had become an insecure bookworm who always thought I was fat regardless of how I looked.

Through my high school years my weight fluctuated continuously and I remained highly insecure about my looks. For much of my life whenever a camera came out I took immediate evasive action. In spite of these insecurities, I had aspirations of being an actress. So I spent time working with a number of local theatre groups.

When I was 21 I moved to New York City. Even though at this time I weighed approximately 150 pounds (which was at least 20 pounds too much), I looked OK, and frequently drew whistles when I walked down the street. It was shortly after I moved to NYC that I went to the doctor on Fifth Avenue who gave me the 600 calorie a day diet which did cause me to lose weight for awhile.

However, even when you look in the mirror and admire your new size 5 body (including thighs that actually don't touch), living on a 600 calorie a day diet is not exactly nirvana.

It was this same doctor who finally (after much begging and pleading on my part) agreed that, although my thyroid tested at the absolute highest end of the "normal" range, perhaps I could use a low dose of thyroid medication to nudge my thyroid function closer to mid-normal range. The doctor prescribed Synthroid, which was then and is still today one of the most widely prescribed hypothyroid medications. Even though Synthroid wasn't the right medication for me (which I didn't know until years later), it did help a bit in the early years, and I finally had a diagnosis of hypothyroidism to take to other specialists who could potentially help me more.

Although I stayed on the 600 calorie a day diet religiously and tortured myself continuously to insure I stayed in size 5 or 7 clothing, since I was still pursuing an acting career most of the women around me were size 2, size 1, size 0, and I still felt fat. In fact at one point in my life I was convinced that I was overweight because I had spent most of my life BELIEVING I was fat. I even tried hypnotherapy, with no positive result, because my weight issues had nothing to do with my mindset OR my eating habits.

Just for the record, I do believe in the power of hypnosis and hypnotherapy to change behavior, if behavior modification is what is called for in your case. So if you are an overeater or your problems stem from actual over consumption of food, or the need for deep motivation to exercise, I can tell you I know a good many people who were helped tremendously by hypnosis or hypnotherapy.

There were a good many years of my life when a piece of pizza, or a hamburger was such a RARE treat that at any point in time I could tell you the date I last had one, even if the last time I had such a forbidden treat was as much as one or two years prior. I could also quote the calorie content and carbohydrate count of hundreds of foods as easily as I remembered the multiplication tables my third grade teacher drilled into us so thoroughly. Does anyone think this is normal? No – it's not, but I'll bet you have similar stories and experiences. Have faith – there is help in these pages.

At the tender age of 30, I got tired of never earning enough to support myself and quit acting. At the same time I decided to modify my diet plan (and quit torturing myself quite so severely), and allowed myself 800 to 900 calories a day.

By age 34, several dozen diets, and several specialists later, I weighed 160. When I stepped on the scales in yet another doctor's office and this was the horrifying calculation from the malicious scale, I panicked and went back on the 600 calorie a day diet until I reached 135 pounds, at which point I was a comfortable size 9.

Let's not forget that over the years, the fashion industry has increased their sizing parameters for women's clothing several times in an effort to make women happier and more secure about their clothing size. Today's "standard" size eight dress would have been marked size eleven in the 1960s. The same dress would have been approximately size ***sixteen*** in the 1940s. So even clothing manufacturers can be construed as being part of the problem that has resulted in over 68% of the US population being overweight.

As usual my weight loss didn't last. I also realized that every time I lost weight, I ultimately gained the weight back and the pounds I gained back would bring along a few extra friends to punish me for having attempted to get rid of them in the first place.

By age 40 I was having serious problems losing even 1 or 2 pounds, and then the following year my weight began inching up slowly but relentlessly. By age 44 it truly didn't matter anymore how little I ate or how much I exercised, my weight inevitably increased, increased, increased, spinning completely out of control and there didn't seem to be anything I could do to stop it. My weight reached 285 pounds by the time I was 52, and hovered there until I was finally properly diagnosed and medicated.

Over the years, I have been to dozens of mainstream doctors and specialists. Nearly all of them told me I had no physical issues causing my ever increasing weight, I simply needed to eat less and exercise more. I love telling these guys I eat one chicken breast and two salads a day, and then having the doctor give me a knowing smirk and a sad shake of the head over my need to lie to them. I have frequently thought there should be some "free pass" form of temporary insanity defense for obese people who punch out a smug, thin doctor – like a "road rage" defense for dieters.

Although I got more empathy and more humane treatment from doctors specializing in alternative medicine, they provided no more productive assistance than their mainstream brethren and, in many cases, came at a much higher price that my insurance didn't cover.

Then there were the occasional doctors who ***did*** believe something was wrong. Some of them were real doozies. I was diagnosed with mercury poisoning and told that since my body was storing the mercury in fat to protect me from the toxin; this was why I couldn't lose weight. I did have high levels of mercury (probably from years of eating a scoop of tuna salad over a bed of dry lettuce for lunch), but after a multi-month, multi-thousand dollar course of twice weekly intravenous chelation treatments, I was free of mercury and still gaining weight.

I have been prescribed $2,000 per month HGH injections for my weight (which my insurance refused to cover) to no avail; been on elaborate vitamin regimes; charted my temperature hourly; charted my blood sugar hourly; and have been subjected to extensive and expensive testing for latent food allergies (which showed I was allergic to several foods I never eat because I don't like them).

I have tried hypnosis, hypnotherapy, sleep learning, brain patterning tapes, neurolinguistic programming, meditation, and exercise programs of virtually every variety from Aqua Aerobics to Zumba.

I have purchased every piece of exercise equipment I have ever seen on an infomercial or in a sporting goods store if it promised I would lose weight while exercising only ten minutes per session three times a week. Shouldn't you lose weight just because you spend the money?

I have purchased at least a 3 month supply of literally every pill for which I have ever received an advertisement by mail promising me I will lose weight. I'm sure you have seen these – an envelope, usually 8 ½ by 6 ½, arrives in the mail with "CONFIDENTIAL" stamped on the outside of it. You open it up, and numerous pieces of paper are inside, including pictures, a newsletter and other fascinating literature about how the ingredients for this pill were discovered by a Swedish doctor secretly working for decades in Machu Piccu or the Amazon Rain Forest, and the magic pills or potion that will miraculously reduce your weight in just 30 days regardless of what you eat or if you never move off your couch, is being fiendishly withheld from us by the FDA. Your money back if it doesn't work is guaranteed.

I admit it – I'm a sucker. I fall for it every time. First I throw it away, telling myself it's just another scam. But then I can't get it out of my head. What if this is the one thing that will make me slender, and I've thrown it away!! What if this doctor really did discover the magic pill and now I'll ***NEVER*** be thin?! In the dead of night when my husband is asleep, I dig the order form out of the trash, fill it out and charge it to my credit card so he won't know how gullible I am. I wait breathlessly for the miracle pills to arrive, and 30 days after that, when the sugar pills they sent me haven't worked at all (again), I find the company has absconded with my money and I've gained three more pounds. If you had any idea how much money I have spent on diet products that didn't work . . . suffice it to say, if I had back all that money I could probably retire.

EUREKA!

Shortly after my 54th birthday I first saw yet another in a long line of doctors who were purportedly brilliant and would help me with my weight problems. With my scale tipping at nearly 285 pounds, I underwent an entire physical, complete with numerous highly specialized tests of my thyroid and adrenal functions.

When the good doctor compassionately began a discussion of gastric by-pass or lap band surgery with me, I had a fit. After hearing me out about the numerous thyroid medications that had ***never*** helped me, and a very spirited, lengthy discussion of what I actually ***DIDN'T*** eat, two things happened. The doctor (who was older and had knowledge of medications before Synthroid), agreed with me when I told him of my research into thyroid medication made from desiccated porcine thyroid and my belief that this would help me. Based on my research, he agreed that we could try a thyroid medication which had been used for over a hundred years, but had fallen out of favor in the 1970's, Armour Thyroid.

Even though I'm pretty sure he didn't believe me when I told him what I usually ate (or ***didn't*** eat), he explained he wanted to have a colleague of his consult with us on managing my diabetes and weight issues.

At my first appointment with the colleague, he didn't believe me at all when I gave him an overview of my normal eating habits. He demanded I keep a food journal, suggesting that most people didn't realize how much they ate until they saw it in writing (yeah, sure). He also insisted I take a diet medication, explaining that the pills weren't ***JUST*** for appetite suppression, they also increased your metabolism which was assistance I clearly needed. Hesitantly I agreed to take a low dose of phentermine. Mind you, I was already on the maximum dose allowable of oral medication for my diabetes, a statin for my cholesterol, meds to regulate my triglycerides and medication for acid reflux, plus my thyroid medication, of course.

After a few months on the new regimen of Armour Thyroid and phentermine, I had lost three pounds! Ok, maybe three pounds in four months isn't exactly something to write home about, but it was the first three pounds I'd actually ***lost*** in more than a decade!

By this point, since I was regularly turning in my food journal (which my husband certified as being correct), ***both*** doctors ***finally believed*** I was eating what I told them I was eating. They brilliantly concluded that there had to be some additional problem that was still undiagnosed. *(YA THINK?!!!)*

Although I had been asked by several doctors over the years if I had ever been diagnosed with sleep apnea, when my response was negative, no one ***ever, EVER,*** followed-up and suggested a sleep study. Approximately six months prior to starting the new medication regimen, I had started seeing an acupuncturist for the first time (also an effort to control my weight), and he had repeatedly asked me about the possibility of sleep apnea. I mentioned this to my new weight loss specialist.

My doctors decided it was time to start ruling out every possibility. They prescribed a sleep study. The results of that sleep study were the turning point of my life.

Many, or perhaps even most, people who have been diagnosed as medically obese or, even worse, morbidly obese are *NOT* necessarily overeating. Regardless of what medical science wants us to believe, I can't make this point often enough. The vast majority of these people have been cursed with bodies that are **NOT** (for whatever reason) properly handling the food they ***DO*** consume, and medical science has failed them.

If the reason you are overweight is that you overeat, or you eat the wrong foods, the answer is simple. **STOP!** If you are overeating for some medical or psychological reason, there is plenty of help available. Many doctors are more than willing to prescribe appetite suppressants for the obese, and therapists specializing in weight reduction therapy techniques can be found on virtually every corner.

I don't mean to trivialize serious psychological problems. I once met a woman who had a case of food addiction so severe it was truly frightening. But look in the yellow pages or online. If you are overeating for whatever reason, help for most people with these types of problems is a phone call and a few blocks away.

If it does *NOT* seem reasonable to believe that you are overweight because of what you eat, it is highly likely that you (like me) have undiagnosed, incorrectly diagnosed, or improperly treated health problems that have nothing to do with what you eat or how much you exercise.

In just a few more pages, we're going to talk about food, and what most of us should be eating or avoiding in order to help ourselves back to a healthy weight. *HOWEVER*, I cannot stress enough, it is crucial for your medical problems to be properly diagnosed and for you to be receiving ***proper*** treatment and/or prescription medications for these health issues that actually resolve them.

You will find extensive information in this book about the most common health issues that can negatively affect your weight or your ability to lose weight. Conditions that are commonly undiagnosed, mis-diagnosed, mis-treated, or about which many doctors will ***never even*** *TELL* you in the first place. This information should help 90% or more of the people that read this book who have been trying to find answers. I can't promise that 100% of people with an undiagnosed medical issue will find their answers in these pages. But I **can** promise that *UNTIL* you are properly medically diagnosed and receiving a treatment or medication that actually resolves your problems, like me, you may never lose weight regardless of what you do, how little you eat, or how much you exercise.

One of the primary purposes of this book is to put the information in your hands that will help you identify your potential medical issues and find a doctor who will diagnose and properly treat those conditions.

WE DON'T NEED NO STINKIN' DIETS

I have spent most of my adult life hoping (praying, actually) that someone would invent the magic pill that would make me thin. The fact of the matter is that ***IF*** the health issues that are preventing your body from properly regulating your weight are finally diagnosed and treated, your body should ***AUTOMATICALLY*** reset itself and magically reduce to what you are ***supposed*** to weigh.

Even though the word "diet" is in the title of this book, (after all, I needed the right people to buy the book) at this point we're going to forget the word "diet."

A "diet" is what the drop dead gorgeous, size 2, perky blonde at the gym goes on when she feels the need to lose the 3 pesky pounds she gained over the holidays. ***A "diet" is something that most people think of as TEMPORARY.***

The changes, small or dramatic, that most of us have to make if our weight problems have continued for years, decades or our entire lives, will be permanent changes. We must form new eating habits that will stay with us for the rest of our lives.

If you only take two things away from this book the most important things are:

1. **The health issues that are preventing your body from correctly regulating your weight must be properly diagnosed and treated.**

2. **You have to map out and design a dining and exercise program that is right for you. One you can live with and stick to for the rest of your life.**

Don't let these statements intimidate you. This book is going to help you achieve your personal goals.

Don't say *"I can't"* – of course you can.

Don't say *"nothing has ever worked before"* – if you hadn't tried and failed before (probably many times just like I have) you wouldn't be reading this book.

What I am talking about is a relationship with food and what you eat that is going to last for a lifetime. Everyone is different, so this program is meant to be ***evolutionary***,

- As you make new discoveries about how certain foods affect your body and your weight, you will want to make changes.
- As your daily schedule fluctuates (your job, your travels, your kids, your responsibilities, your life) you will need to make changes.
- As new information becomes available, you will want to make changes.

Meeting these criteria requires a program that is flexible, allowing you to be in charge of what you eat. Forget the word "diet". That word no longer exists for us.

We are talking about:

DYNAMIC DINING DESIGN!

- ***Dynamic*** because it is flexible and evolutionary. Immediately adaptable at all times to meet your changing needs.
- ***Dining*** because to dine implies a different relationship with food than merely eating or choking down something tasteless that does nothing more than fill a nutritional requirement.
- ***Design*** is obvious. You design it yourself to meet your specifications, your needs and your preferences.

Dynamic Dining Design is a way of life that will result in a whole new you. You are going to let the healthy person inside you out. You are going to be amazed at how easy and pleasurable it will be to dine on actual food that tastes good, which satisfies your body and your mind and your taste buds, and yet keeps you trim and fit, the way your body was meant to be.

You must also recognize that mapping out **your PERSONAL** ***Dynamic Dining Design program*** will be an evolutionary process. You cannot expect to get it 100% right the first time. That's OK! The important things are:

- Start with a design and as you go along, tweak things that don't work for you.
- Forgive yourself if you fall off the wagon. Don't chuck the whole plan and all your hard work just

because you had a fight with your boyfriend, husband, BFF, boss, ***whoever***, and ate an entire pint of Rocky Road. Get up the next morning, look in the mirror and tell yourself you know you F****d up, forgive yourself, and get back to your **personal** ***Dynamic Dining Design program***. Too many people chuck the whole thing just because of one little stumble.

- Be kind to yourself. Just don't make a habit of stumbling off your path every other day.

Before mapping out your personal Dynamic Dining Design program, here are some basic guidelines:

ONE: ESSENTIAL EDIBLES. First and foremost, there are certain foods that will be completely individual to you that are impossible for you to give up.

If you try to design a Dynamic Dining Design program that leaves out these ***Essential Edibles*** completely, you will ***NEVER*** be successful because you are being onerous to yourself, punishing yourself, and you will fall off your program big time. On the plus side, you will give yourself the satisfaction of chalking up one more diet failure in your martyrdom. You won't hurt anyone but yourself, and nobody loves a martyr. Trust me.

To figure out what Essential Edible items are most important to you, you have to think about what you can't get through a day or a week without. **THIS CANNOT BE A LONG LIST.** But if there are one or two or a ***MAXIMUM*** of three Essential Edibles, foods or beverages you cannot live without, now is the time to figure out what those are so you can design your personal Dynamic Dining Design program around them.

For me, my number one Essential Edible is wine. If I can't have a glass or two of wine with dinner, at least a couple of times a week, life just isn't worth living. Obviously this has nothing to do with drinking, because one or two glasses of wine never got anyone drunk – or even tipsy for most people. I love the ritual and the elegance and the taste of wine. If you're a Star Trek fan you may remember Diana and the Chocolate Ice Cream Sundae from Star Trek Second Generation – the way she felt about chocolate is how I feel about wine.

From the ritual of opening the bottle with a nice corkscrew (don't ask me to drink wine from a bottle with a screw on cap), to pouring that first soupçon in the glass to establish the wine is good, swirling the wine around and holding it up to the light to see the shimmer of the color and clarity of the legs – to that first sip as the taste of the wine bursts across your tongue and the complex flavors tickle your palate – for me it is about the taste and the luxury of the experience. It makes me feel decadent and luxurious and pampered.

Of course, if Crystal Light came out tomorrow with a flavor that replicated (down to the last lingering note) the taste of the wine I love, I'd save the calories and drink that. But until that happens, I just have to suck it up and give up other stuff in favor of the occasional glass of wine.

Second for me is macaroni and cheese. I don't have to have it all the time – or even often, but once every six or eight weeks I have to work in a reasonable size portion of my favorite comfort food.

If I have a number three it's probably pizza – but that's a distant third for me. If I have a couple of slices of pizza once every three or four months I'm usually happy.

You have to decide what your Essential Edibles are. Whether its beer, or chocolate or good scotch, or a bagel, or cheesecake, or pasta primavera, if you don't work these two or three things into your Dynamic Dining Design program on an infrequent but regular basis of some sort, you're just setting yourself up for failure.

TWO: EXERCISE. A close second in the basics, is Regular Exercise (yes, the dreaded Regular Exercise).

You must have some exercise in your life, and it must be something you will actually do religiously three or four times a week. You must choose something you enjoy (or at least don't hate) that you absolutely will do, because again, if you choose something you hate, and you view your chosen exercise as a punishment, you will find every reason in the world not to do it. (Believe me, I'm the Queen of excuses.)

First of all, it should be fun. I know, exercise fun? But it truly can be. Dancing is excellent exercise, as is skating of any kind, or even tai chi.

Second, it ***MUST*** fit into your routine. For instance, if you travel all the time and you need a bunch of special equipment to do your chosen exercise, you have set yourself up for failure and you won't do it. So whatever you choose must fit into your routine, your lifestyle and your budget. If you are having trouble coming up with a good exercise plan, walking is always the best, simplest and easiest exercise and you can do it absolutely anywhere on the planet. If necessary you can walk in circles in a room.

Third, if you are anywhere close to as overweight as I was, the exercise cannot be too strenuous. Whatever you choose, if you can only do it for five minutes starting out, only do it for five minutes. Don't let anyone make you feel guilty either. You know what you can do and if you push yourself beyond what you can do, you'll just stop doing it. When you are ready to go to seven minutes, go to seven minutes, it doesn't matter if it's one month or six months before you increase the time. What matters is that you are exercising on a regular (three or four times a week) basis. You know what you can do, and if you don't do as much exercise as you could or should, you're only hurting yourself. But remember, the goal is 30 minutes of exercise four times a week even if it takes you a year to get there!

> Next, you must consider location. For some people having a place to go and participating with others doing the same exercise is both necessary and a fun social outlet. Some may choose a personal trainer or another type of structure. For others, exercise in any form is a solitary pursuit. For instance, I have to design an exercise plan that I can do at home – from both the perspective of fitting the exercise into my daily routine as well my personal preferences, exercise is something I only do alone.
>
> If you enjoy jazzercise classes or other classes at your local dance studio, join the class of your choice. If you enjoy going to the gym, by all means, go.

Personally, I view a gym with the same level of enthusiasm that I view the seven circles of Dante's Hell. Even if I steel myself to go in and join the gym, once I get there I have to listen to the perky size zero blonde with an IQ of 2 wearing the hot pink and turquoise leotard with (oh my god) HORIZONTAL stripes that make her look great (and would make me look like a fashion disaster from the whale section), tell me about the joys of the gym and how much weight I will lose. And let's not forget her hunky compatriot, in the tank top that's five sizes too small and the short shorts that show off his butt, who waxes poetic (or as poetic as a guy with more biceps than brains can achieve) about how caring and attentive the trainers are. Eventually, I let myself actually be intimidated or shamed into plunking down my credit card for the exorbitant membership fee plus the one year monthly contract payments . . . (hummm, I guess the blonde and the hunk aren't quite as dumb as I think since they just earned a hefty commission) . . . knowing I am going to hate myself.

After this occurs, with my credit limit now severely depleted, ***IF*** I actually convince myself to pack up my gym bag with all the accoutrement and go to the gym to exercise, it's a miracle.

When I get to the gym and slink quietly in the front door, it seems that all activity stops and an unnatural silence descends as I walk up to the treadmill area where everyone else is running perkily while simultaneously texting and sipping a health smoothie. There I am in my 5X oversized tee shirt that's supposed to hide the fat (oh sure, no one would ever guess it's all me under there), and my spandex pants – standing there like a dork trying to figure out how to program the damn treadmill. Of course, everyone else pretends not to see me, because fat might be contagious . . . and all the supposedly compassionate trainers ignore me in favor of – (the gay ones) other hunks who are charmingly clumsy, or – (the straight ones) the perky size 2 women who might break a nail operating their PDA.

It's at this point I usually run (don't walk) for a cab and, the minute my apartment door slams behind me, break out a magnum of wine and a pint of Cherry Garcia. After all, if I give my cats kitty treats they will sit with me and commiserate and Ryan Seacrest can make me forget my blues after enough of the wine has been consumed.

Meanwhile the gym has — ***Ka-Ching!!*** — cashed in on yet another sucker who plunked down several thousand dollars and will never darken their doorway again.

As I said earlier, it's important to choose an exercise plan that is appropriate for you.

DYNAMIC DINING DESIGN

The ***Dynamic Dining Design*** program is strategically engineered to last a lifetime. It provides ultimate flexibility, allowing you to make choices that fit your preferences, your lifestyle, the time you have to allocate to food/meal planning, and what you actually ***LIKE*** to eat. The more you are able to include foods you like to eat, the greater the chance that you will be successful with the program and that it will become your lifelong routine, comfortable as an old pair of jeans. This program is guaranteed to allow your body to achieve your perfect weight.

I'm going to repeat here information from the prior chapter. For those of you who didn't read "We Don't Need No Stinkin' Diets" and (like me) skipped straight to the chapter with the program, please GO BACK and read AT LEAST this one chapter. It has some essential information in it. However, to repeat, why ***DYNAMIC DINING DESIGN?***

- ***Dynamic*** because it is flexible and evolutionary. Immediately adaptable at all times to meet your changing needs.
- ***Dining*** because to dine implies a different relationship with food than merely eating or choking down something tasteless that does nothing more than fill a nutritional requirement.
- ***Design*** is obvious. You design it yourself to meet your specifications, your needs and your preferences.

I'm told by some of my friends that it is easier for them to stick with a new eating routine, at least in the beginning, if they have been given structure and are *NOT* given the freedom to make their own choices its easier for them. If this is YOUR preference, you will find a set of sample menus in Appendix 5 which can be utilized until you get the hang of the Dynamic Dining Design program and feel more comfortable taking advantage of the built-in flexibility.

Dynamic Dining Design is a very simple program that is easy to follow. **However, it is essential that you pay attention to what is ALLOWED and what is *BUDGETED or FORBIDDEN.***

Over the course of time it will not be necessary to strictly count calories or carbohydrates. However, when you first start the program it is important to keep a food journal along with a running total of the calories and carbohydrates you consume each day. I'd suggest you keep the food journal for at least six months, until you reach the point that keeping mental track of what you are eating becomes second nature. The food journal will also be extremely useful in helping you identify how certain foods affect your ability to lose weight.

Once you are convinced that any and all health issues that have previously stopped your body from positively regulating your weight are being successfully treated *and YOU ARE REGULARLY LOSING WEIGHT*, then it will no longer be as important to keep the food journal.

As long as you are following the Dynamic Dining Design program and sticking to **Allowed** foods, you will continue losing weight until you get to the right weight for your body.

THE DYNAMIC DINING DESIGN PROGRAM

Total Daily Calories:

Recommended for Women	1200 to 1800 MAXIMUM: 2200
Recommended for Men	1500 to 2200 MAXIMUM: 2800

Total Daily Carbohydrates: Recommended: 20-25
MAXIMUM 40

MEALS

Breakfast:

- 2 cups coffee, tea, or other Carte Blanche Beverage
- 1 egg *(see cooking options)*
- 3 ounces Carte Blanche Protein *(see list)*
    - OR 1 additional egg
- Optional: ½ Whole Grain English Muffin

IF you CANNOT EAT EGGS, SUBSTITUTE A TOTAL OF 6 OUNCES PROTEIN (Cheese is an option)

Lunch:

- Salad w/dressing *(see salad and dressing options)*
- 6 ounces Carte Blanche Protein *(broiled or grilled)*
    - OR Soup &1 Protein Salad choice
- ½ cup Carte Blanche Vegetables

Dinner:

- Salad w/dressing *(see salad and dressing options)*
- 8 ounces Carte Blanche Protein *(broiled or grilled)*
- Unlimited Carte Blanche Vegetables

Snacks:

- 2 per day, when most convenient *(see options)*

IF you prefer eating your heavier meal at mid-day, it is perfectly acceptable to flip the Lunch and Dinner menus.

However, it is ***CRITICAL*** to ***EAT BREAKFAST***, as laid out, ***WITHIN 60 MINUTES of GETTING UP each morning***. You will understand the importance of this better after reading about Circadian Rhythm further along in the book.

Now, let's get into the details.

BEVERAGES

NOTES:

- *ALL allowed beverages MUST be sugar free*
- *Beverages may ONLY be sweetened with zero calorie, sugar free, artificial sweeteners*
- *ONLY items from the list of Allowed Condiments or Allowed Miscellaneous may be utilized to alter the taste of Allowed Beverages.*

CARTE BLANCHE BEVERAGES

- Water (plain or sparkling, unflavored, sugar free) the more the better.
- Water, Flavored (Plain or sparkling, zero calorie)
- Mineral Water (plain or sparkling, zero calorie)
- Coffee (sugar free – with or without milk OR artificial (sugar free) creamer)
- Tea (sugar free – all varieties including black, green, and herbal)
- Lemon Press (freshly squeezed lemon and plain or sparkling water)
- Lime Press (freshly squeezed lime and plain or sparkling water)
- Lemon Juice

- Lime Juice
- Grapefruit Juice
- Diet Soda (Sugar free, calorie free, any variety)
- Powdered Drink Mixes (sugar free, calorie free, any variety)
- Bottled/Canned Beverages (sugar free, calorie free, all varieties)

BUDGETED BEVERAGES

- Milk – Limit ½ cup per day. Recommend Skim Plus milk, as that variety of milk tastes like whole milk and acts like whole milk in coffee or tea, but has the benefits of skim milk.
- Half & Half for coffee or tea. Actually better for you than milk. Limit ¼ cup of Half & Half per cup of coffee or tea.
- Vegetable Juice – 1 glass (8 oz) per day from Allowed Vegetable list. No added sugar of any kind. No additives that add calories or carbohydrates. Freshly juiced is best.
- Fruit Juice (Other than Lemon/Lime) – Limit 2 glasses (8 oz ea) per week. ***EXCEPTION:*** 100% natural cranberry juice with no artificial sweeteners or flavorings (Oceanspray does **NOT** fit these requirements) – 7 glasses per week of this type of cranberry juice is permitted.

- Wine – Limit 2 glasses per night, 3 nights per week.
- Beer – Limit 3 regular beers per week. 5 beers permitted if lite beer is chosen.
- Vodka (Unflavored), Tequila, Rum, Gin, Scotch – Limit 8 shots per week.
- Other Alcoholic Beverages – Limit 4 shots per week.
    - A Note about alcoholic beverages – alcohol of any kind can be detrimental to weight loss generally. If drinking alcoholic beverages, be careful to observe how such beverages affect your personal weight loss.

FORBIDDEN BEVERAGES

- Cocktails (due to high sugar content of most cocktails)
- Sherry
- Cordials
- Aperitifs
- Chocolate flavored beverages of any kind
- *Basically any beverage that is NOT on the Carte Blanche or Budgeted list is a forbidden beverage, unless it is sugar free, calorie free, and carbohydrate free. If you*

know of any that were left off the Carte Blanche Beverage list, please let us know.

EGGS

Eggs are one of the most perfect foods you can eat. Because eggs are so special and so amazingly good for you, eggs are being treated as their own separate category. More good nutrition is packed inside that shell that most people even begin to understand. Approximately 70 calories, and 5 grams of fat that is GOOD for you, eggs are one of nature's most perfect foods. Unless you despise eggs, or have some excellent reason for not eating eggs (such as allergies, or religious considerations), I would suggest that you eat 1 or 2 eggs at breakfast every morning.

Medical science has finally admitted that people with high cholesterol ***HAVE*** high cholesterol for reasons ***unrelated*** to eating foods that contain cholesterol (such as eggs). In fact, high cholesterol has proven to be a symptom or side effect of numerous health disorders that have nothing to do with whether or not you consume foods containing cholesterol. So there is no reason to avoid eggs, unless your doctor has specified some other medical reason why you should not have them.

Eggs should be eaten as intended by nature, white, yolk, and all. In fact, much of the nutritional value of an egg is in the yolk.

Eggs referenced in this book are regular chicken's eggs. People eat all kinds of other eggs, and that is fine. Just be aware that other types of eggs, such as duck eggs, goose eggs, turkey eggs, etc, have higher calorie and fat content than chicken eggs. That is not necessarily a bad thing, but you may have to adjust accordingly.

COOKING OPTIONS FOR EGGS

- Boiled (soft or hard, as you prefer)
- Poached

THE ABOVE are the two BEST, most highly preferred cooking methods, as no additional calories or fat are added while cooking.

- Scrambled or fried eggs should be made ***ONLY*** in a non-stick pan utilizing only one pat of butter or a teaspoon (at most) of any allowed oil you prefer.

PROTEIN

CARTE BLANCHE PROTEIN

- **BEEF** (Lean cuts only)
  - Filet Mignon
  - London Broil
  - Top or bottom Round
  - Eye of Round
  - Tenderloin
  - Flank Steak

  - Skirt Steak
  - Sirloin Steak (well trimmed)
  - Cubed Stew Meat
  - Deli Roast Beef *(no sugar added)*
  - Ground Beef/Hamburger *(lean ground)*
- Buffalo/Bison (steaks or burgers)
- Bear
- Veal (all cuts, well trimmed)
- Venison
- Liver (Any)
- Sweet breads
- Rabbit
- Pork Tenderloin
- Sopressata *(no sugar added)*
- Deli Ham *(lean, no sugar added)*
- Knockwurst *(no sugar added)*
- Liverwurst *(no sugar added)*
- Center Cut Pork Chop
- Canadian Bacon *(no sugar added)*
- Lamb Leg
- Lamb Shoulder
- Lamb chops

- Pepperoni *(no sugar added)*
- Salami *(no sugar added)*
- Snake
- Alligator
- **POULTRY**
    - Chicken (light or dark)
    - Turkey (light or dark)
    - Deli Turkey *(no sugar added)*
    - Cornish hen
    - Duck
    - Ostrich
    - Game birds
- **FISH/SEAFOOD**
    - Tuna steak (any variety of tuna)
    - Tuna (canned light in water)
    - Skip Jack Tuna
    - Salmon
    - Arctic Char
    - Whitefish
    - Bluefish
    - Sole
    - Trout
    - Tilapia

- Red Snapper
- Mahi-mahi
- Halibut
- Haddock
- Flounder
- Black Cod (Sablefish)
- Cod
- Carp
- Catfish
- Bass
- Mackerel
- Butterfish
- Orange Roughy
- Turbot
- Perch
- Pike
- Abalone
- Oysters
- Conch
- Clams
- Lobster
- Crab *(real crab ONLY,* ***NO*** *imitation)*
- Shrimp

- Scallops
- Mussels
- Crawfish
- Octopus
- Squid

BUDGETED PROTEINS

- Cold Cuts and luncheon meats not specifically listed (all varieties, Limit 2 servings per week)
- **BEEF**
  - Rib eye or Porterhouse steak (Limit 2 per week)
  - Brisket of beef or spare ribs (Limit 2 per month)
- **PORK**
  - Bacon (lean cut – Limit 3 slices, 3 times per week)
  - Sausage (Limit – 2 links, 3 times per week)
- **POULTRY**
  - Goose (Limit – 1 time per month)
  - Pate or Pate du fois grois (Limit – 1 per month)

FORBIDDEN PROTEIN

- Barbecue beef or pork
- Barbecue ribs
- Any meat or deli meat that contains added sugar
- Anything that is NOT on the ALLOWED list

CHEESE* & DAIRY

CARTE BLANCHE CHEESE & DAIRY

- Plain yogurt (no sugar, no flavorings)
- Tofu
- Cottage cheese (½ cup, plain or mixed with allowed vegetables)
- Very hard cheeses (e.g. Parmesan and Romano)
- Hard cheeses (e.g. Cheddar, Colby, Edam, Gouda, and Swiss)
- Semi-soft cheeses (e.g. American, Bleu, Feta, Havarti, Monterrey Jack, Muenster, Emmenthaler, Gruyere, Gorgonzola, Stilton, Pepper Jack, Provolone)
- Soft cheeses (e.g. Cream Cheese, Ricotta, Mozzarella)
- Cream/Whipped Cream/Sour Cream *(no sugar added)*

- Butter (natural butter, NOT margarine)

BUDGETED CHEESE & DAIRY

- Very soft cheeses (e.g. Brie, Camembert, Port Salut, Borsin, etc.)

  (Limit – 2 times per week)

FORBIDDEN CHEESE & DAIRY

- Anything NOT on the ALLOWED list above

Regular milk (and even skim milk) contains a significant amount of NATURAL sugar. Interestingly, most cheese does not contain sugar, natural or otherwise. When purchasing dairy products, read labels carefully. For instance, the Half and Half I use has LESS THAN 1 Carb per cup, but this varies from product to product. Cream has far less sugar (or no sugar) occurring naturally.

**Cheese counts as a protein and may be substituted for protein.*

SALAD INGREDIENTS

CARTE BLANCHE SALAD INGREDIENTS

- Lettuce (any kind you prefer)
- Spinach

- Cabbage (green or red)
- Watercress
- Mache
- Mescaline greens
- Sorrel
- Arugula
- Escarole
- Chicory
- Sprouts (all varieties)
- Celery
- Cilantro
- Cucumber
- Endive
- Fennel
- Jicama
- Kohlrabi
- Mushrooms
- Onion
- Parsley
- Peppers (all colors)
- Radishes

- Rhubarb
- Scallions
- Seaweed and Sea Vegetables (Nori, etc.)
- Shallots
- Tomato
- Water Chestnut
- Olives
- Avocado

PROTEIN SALADS

- You may add things from other allowed lists (such as cheese, chicken, or shrimp) to your salad, but if adding proteins to salad, you must count the additions as part or all of your protein serving for that meal.

SALAD DRESSING

- Lemon juice plus 1 tbsp. olive or avocado oil
- Vinegar of any kind plus 1 tbsp. olive or avocado oil
- Any packaged dressing with no or very little sugar, salad spritzers are very good choices

FORBIDDEN SALAD INGREDIENTS

- Croutons
- Pasta of any kind
- Snow peas
- Squash of any kind
- Anything NOT on the ALLOWED Salad or Vegetable list

VEGETABLES

CARTE BLANCHE VEGETABLES

- Asparagus
- Bamboo shoots
- Bok choi
- Broccoli or broccoli rabe
- Brussels sprouts
- Cabbage (green or red)
- Cauliflower
- Celery
- Dark leafy green vegetables (Kale, spinach, etc.)
- Leeks
- Okra

- Green beans
- Chard
- Chick peas
- Chicory
- Collard greens
- Mustard greens
- Kale
- Fennel
- Escarole
- Corn
- Lentils
- Mushrooms
- Parsnip
- Celery root (Celeriac)
- Turnip greens

FORBIDDEN VEGETABLES

- All starchy vegetables (e.g. peas, lotus root, carrots)
- Eggplant
- Squash of all varieties
- Peas and snow peas

- Beans not otherwise listed
- Lima beans and butter beans

CONDIMENTS

CARTE BLANCHE CONDIMENTS

- Lemon juice
- Lime juice
- Vinegar (all varieties)
- Pepper (all colors)
- Soy sauce (note: soy negatively affects thyroid)
- Mustard (yellow, brown or Dijon)
- Tabasco sauce
- Worcestershire sauce
- Chilies or hot peppers
- All herbs (any variety)
- All spices (any variety)
- Extracts (vanilla, almond, etc.)
- Horse radish *(NO added sugar)*
- Hot sauces *(NO added sugar)*
- Olive oil
- Avocado Oil

- Coconut Oil
- Salsa *(NO added sugar)*
- Salt (sea salt recommended)
- Wasabi
- Mayonnaise *(NO added sugar)*
- Garlic
- Ginger
- Butter (real butter NOT margarine)
- Nut oils
- Organic vegetable oils
- Any 0 calorie artificial sweetener

FORBIDDEN CONDIMENTS

- Ketchup
- Teriyaki Sauce
- Steak sauce
- Barbecue sauce
- Corn Oil

MISCELLANEOUS

CARTE BLANCHE MISCELLANEOUS

- Broth – beef, poultry or vegetable *(NO added sugar)*
- Soups (*with no added sugars*, and the ingredients do ***not*** contain anything that is NOT allowed)
- Yogurt (Unflavored, Sugar free, no fruit added. Plain and/or Greek yogurt is best)
- Hummus
- Edamame
- Popcorn
- Grapefruit
- Pickles (all varieties with NO sugar and >1 Carb per oz)
- Nuts (Almonds, pistachios, cashews and walnuts are especially good)
- Chia Seeds
- Other Fiber Supplements *(no sugar added)*

BUDGETED MISCELLANEOUS

- Honey (Limit 2 Tblspn per week)
- Potatoes (Limit 1 per week. Baked, Grilled or Roasted)

- Wraps (tortilla wraps for sandwiches)
- Japanese sticky rice (in very limited quantities when eating sushi)
- Long grain wild rice (2 times per month)
- Apples (Limit 1 per week)
- Watermelon (Limit 2 times per month)
- Banana (Limit 2 per month)
- FRUITS (Limit 1 cup per month from all Budgeted fruit this means 1 cup ONLY, NOT 1 cup of each item)
    - Cherries
    - Cranberries
    - Blueberries
    - Blackberries
    - Raspberries
    - Grapes
    - Oranges
    - Strawberries
    - Plums

FORBIDDEN MISCELLANEOUS

- Bread of any kind NOT on the allowed list
- Fruit of any kind NOT on the allowed list

- Trail mix
- Starches of any kind NOT on the allowed list
- Pasta
- Basically ANYTHING **NOT** on the ALLOWED list is FORBIDDEN.

SNACKS

- Small salad
- 1.5 oz Carte Blanche Cheese with unlimited Celery Sticks
- Quarter cup of nuts
- ½ avocado (mashed) with 1 piece cheddar cheese melted over it
- 3 oz Yogurt (sugar free, no fruit added)
- 2 oz Hummus on Endive Leaves or Celery Sticks
- 2 oz Nut Butter on Endive Leaves, Celery Sticks, or Rhubarb Sticks.
- 1.5 oz Turkey Breast rolled with lettuce and Carte Blanche Condiment of your choice
- 1.5 oz Carte Blanche Protein rolled with lettuce and Carte Blanche Condiment of your choice
- 4 oz any Carte Blanche Vegetable
- 4 oz Beef, Poultry, or Vegetable broth

- 3 oz Edamame
- Small bowl popcorn
- Half small grapefruit

COOKING OPTIONS

PROTEINS

- Broiled
- Grilled
- Roasted
- Baked
- Boiled (if appropriate)
- Sautéed (in a small amount of butter or your choice of allowed oil)

VEGETABLES

- Raw is always the best way to preserve the greatest nutritional value
- Steamed
- Microwaved
- Boiled (this cooking method depletes vitamin and fiber benefits of many vegetables)

- Sautéed (in a small amount of butter or your choice of allowed oil. OR use beef or chicken broth or bullion to sauté)
- Stir Fried
- Grilled (grilling brings out wonderful flavors in most vegetables)
- Roasted in a closed clay casserole in the oven (this cooking method intensifies the flavor of many vegetables, and is absolutely delicious)

TIPS, NOTES, and IMPORTANT INFORMATION

- **FORGET EVERYTHING** you think you already know about weight loss. This is a new way of life. You cannot compare ***Dynamic Dining Design*** to any other weight loss program you have ever read or tried.
- ***Dynamic Dining Design*** IS FLEXIBLE TO SUIT YOUR LIFESTYLE. If you prefer to cook meals from scratch all the time, knock yourself out. Alternatively, eat all the pre-packaged or microwave foods you want if that suits your lifestyle. OR eat out all the time if you prefer; even McDonalds has salads these days.
- As previously noted, counting calories and carbs is not strictly necessary. But it is important to get used to the portion size you should be eating of the right foods.
    - Portion size is something you may have to experiment with.

- ✓ Basically eat until you aren't hungry, and STOP. ***BUT*** be aware that your body won't TELL YOU that you're NOT hungry until 10 to 15 minutes AFTER you have eaten a sufficient quantity of food.
- ✓ Learn to end your meal after eating the right portions and trust that you have eaten the correct amount.
- ✓ The right portion for me won't be the right portion for you and certainly won't be the right portion for Jane.

- PURCHASE A KITCHEN FOOD SCALE. Until you become familiar with appropriate serving sizes, use the food scale.
  - BUTCHERS ARE HAPPY TO HELP. Even in giant supermarket chains, most butchers are willing to break open packages of fresh meat and poultry and do the work of weighting and cutting portions to the appropriate sizes for you. They will also trim meats even leaner if you request.
- If you are following the food lists and staying within the Carte Blanche items, it doesn't really matter if you count anything, so long as you are eating 3 reasonable meals and 2 reasonable snacks each day.
  - The food lists make this diet simple.
    - ✓ Eat what's on the lists.
    - ✓ **Don't** eat what's *NOT* on the list.

- DINE ON A FAIRLY REGULAR SCHEDULE if possible. It will help to keep you from getting hungry and potentially overeating. Your body will "learn" the schedule and you will find you get hungry when you normally eat.
- **BREAKFAST IS CRITICAL!** If you cannot eat all your meals on a schedule, ***AT LEAST EAT YOUR BREAKFAST WITHIN 60 MINUTES OF GETTING UP.*** This is very important; as you will understand once you have read about circadian rhythms and sleep problems later in the book.
- It is best to finish your food for the day no later than 9:00 pm if possible.
- Always eat your salad first at lunch and dinner, and drink plenty of any allowed beverage. This will get the healthiest, lowest calorie food into your system first and reduce your hunger, which should reduce the overall amount you consume during a meal.
- EXERCISE AT RANDOM TIMES if possible. You can force your body to burn more calories by exercising at random times from day to day. It has been shown that if you exercise at the same time every day, your body "remembers" your schedule, and compensates for the daily exercise by burning fewer calories during the period you regularly exercise.
    - EXERCISE AT LEAST 3 to 4 times a week.
    - EXERCISE GOAL IS 30 MINUTES per exercise session. Try to work up to 30 minutes per session no matter how long it takes to work up to this goal.

- DRINK PLENTY OF FLUIDS. Drink water (best) or other Carte Blanche beverages. It is important to drink plenty of liquids to flush your system regularly and insure you are always adequately hydrated (which will help you lose weight). Additionally, drinking plenty of fluids will help you feel less hungry.
- ***Dynamic Dining Design*** is a common sense approach to high protein, low carbohydrate dieting. There are numerous reasons for this, which you will understand as you read the rest of this book.
    - It is a scientific fact that people on high protein, low carbohydrate weight loss programs loose nearly twice as much weight as people on other types of programs.
    - Protein, especially lean protein, builds muscle.
    - Protein promotes thermo genesis. This process causes your body to naturally burn fat.
    - Protein is burned slower by your body than carbohydrates. This means you won't get hungry as often and your energy levels will remain consistent.
    - Protein makes people feel more satisfied, and satisfaction is essential to weight loss.
- It's true that the calorie range goes from 1200 for a small woman to 2800 for a man. If you are a tall man and need 2500 calories a day, eat a slightly larger portion of protein, add chopped egg or shredded cheese to your salads. Regardless of calories ALWAYS stick with less than 40 carbs per day.

- PLAN FOR YOUR MEALS. This does not mean you must spend hours cooking and shopping (I don't have time for that either). But even if you are just going to microwave something or eat a salad, it is better to know what you plan to eat and insure it is available at the appropriate time, than to find yourself hungry two hours past the time you should have eaten and discover you have no allowed food in the house.

- EATING SHOULD NOT BE BORING. Studies have shown that people tend to restrict themselves to the same limited group of about 15 to 20 foods all the time. DO NOT restrict yourself; there are numerous allowed foods to choose from. Variety is the spice of live, so live it up.

- **ALWAYS USE ARTIFICIAL SWEETNERS**. Never add sugar to anything. If purchasing pre-packaged food or eating at a restaurant, always choose non-sweetened everything over anything that contains sugar of any kind.

    - Artificial Sweeteners are ***NOT*** created equally (no pun intended). Here is the brief low-down on artificial sweeteners. You will have to decide which artificial sweetener is right for you. Any will do, as long as they are FREE of calories and carbohydrates.

        - ✓ Saccharine is my favorite artificial sweetener. It has been available since about 1880. It has zero calories, zero carbohydrates, and is safe for diabetics. It is approximately 300 times sweeter than sugar and doesn't change when heated, so it works well in tea, coffee, or other hot foods/beverages. The 1970s cancer scare regarding saccharine was greatly exaggerated, and medical science now admits there is no scientific correlation between saccharine and cancer in humans.

- ✓ Aspartame is also a calorie-free option that is safe for diabetics. Aspartame is approximately 200 times sweeter than sugar. It does break down with heat, so using it in hot beverages or food is not recommended.

- ✓ Sucralose is actually chemically altered sugar. It has no calories. Sucralose is approximately 600 times sweeter than sugar, but it holds up in heat and can be used freely in hot beverages and foods. Some people have reported abdominal discomfort when using Sucralose.

- ✓ Stevia is an all-natural, zero calorie sweetener derived from the leaf of the stevia plant. You can use Stevia in hot beverages and foods; however it does best in only medium hot temperatures. While the FDA has declared Stevia to be safe, it has been recommended by the Mayo Clinic that it should only be used in moderation. Consult your doctor before use if you are pregnant.

- DO NOT BE INTIMIDATED IN RESTAURANTS. Never be afraid to give the waiter specific instructions regarding how you want your food presented:
    - Broiled, not fried
    - Sauces on the side
    - ***Salad dressing ALWAYS on the sid***e, so you can control the portion
    - DO NOT ALLOW STARCH on your plate. If the starch comes automatically with the meal, refuse it. Tell them to leave the starch in the kitchen. If something is on your plate, you will be much more tempted to eat it than if it is NOT THERE.
    - SUBSTITUTE what you want for what you don't want if the restaurant allows it (green beans rather than rice; extra broccoli rather than pasta). I rarely eat in restaurants that DO NOT allow substitutions. I always offer to pay extra, if necessary, for the substitution.
    - Telling the wait staff you are ALLERGIC to whatever you do not want will result in IMMEDIATE compliance with your instructions, and should result in allowing substitutes even in restaurants that say they do not allow substitutions. Every restaurant is highly concerned with legal liabilities surrounding allergic reactions.

Remember the movie, "When Harry Met Sally?" When that movie came out dozens of friends called me to ask which of the writers knew me – this was because of the way Sally ordered in restaurants throughout the movie. IF THEY DON'T BRING YOUR FOOD THE WAY YOU ORDERED IT, SEND IT BACK.

- Full fat cheese is good for you. In research published in the Annals of Internal Medicine, it was shown that people with high levels of trans-palmitoleic acid (a compound found in dairy fat) were 60% less likely to develop Type 2 Diabetes than those with the lowest levels. This compound has also been linked with being at a healthy weight.
- There is nothing wrong with eating fat, as long as you eat the RIGHT KINDS of fat. There is NO NEED to avoid fat like the plague, and, as you can see, fat is certainly included and allowed in the program. However, use common sense. Do NOT eat butter a stick at a time or consume olive oil by the cup.
    - Healthy Fats include:
        - ✓ Saturated fats are solid at room temperature. They are a stable type of fat, and are fine to eat. Saturated fats include most animal fat, although mono-saturated fats are the healthiest.
        - ✓ Fat contains 9 calories per gram.
        - ✓ The BEST sources of healthy fat are olive oil, avocado oil, butter (NEVER MARGARINE), and the Omega-3 fatty acids founds in many types of fish.
        - ✓ Fats that are known as Essential Fatty Acids include Omega-3 and Omega-6

fats. Omega-6 fats are found in nuts and vegetable oils.

- ✓ Olive oil, avocado oil, nuts, and nut oils are excellent sources of mono-saturated fat.
- ✓ In Italy vast quantities of olive oil are consumed by one and all. Italy also has the lowest rate of cardiovascular disease of anywhere on earth.

- o **UN**-healthy Fats include:
  - ✓ Poly-UNsaturated fat is an UNstable fat. This type of fat carries large quantities of free radicals. Free radicals promote plaque in the arteries and could be a cause of high cholesterol. These types of fat are linked to insulin resistance and high triglycerides.
  - ✓ Trans-fats and Trans-Fatty Acids are also unhealthy types of fat. Unless a label clearly states "No Trans-Fats" OR "No Trans-Fatty Acids", you should assume that most processed and fried foods, and MOST MARGERINE contains these types of fat.

- Never consume Fake Fats, such as OLESTRA. Artificial fillers designed to make food more palatable are also to be avoided. Both Fake Fats and Artificial Fillers can actually inhibit weight loss.
- Margarine is much more harmful than butter. You should never eat margarine. In 1995 the Harvard

Nurses Study showed a higher incidence of cardiovascular disease from eating margarine than butter.

- **READ LABELS, READ LABELS, READ LABELS**. This is so critical, I cannot stress how very important it is to read labels and insure you know what is in your food. Regardless of whether everything you eat is cooked lovingly from scratch, OR whether everything you eat comes out of the microwave or from a restaurant, ***YOU MUST KNOW WHAT IS IN YOUR FOOD***. There are tons of unnecessary hidden sugars and fake fat in many foods that will slow down weight loss. There are also many other things that are not good for your weight in some foods, especially packaged ready-to-serve foods. You will be surprised more often than you can imagine as to what is in there if you carefully read food labels.

- Canned vegetables (or any other food) are fine if this is what suits your lifestyle, but again, READ LABELS. Make sure your vegetables do NOT have added sugar. The label of the canned Green String Beans I prefer indicates the ingredients are: "Green String Beans, Water, and Salt." Period.

- Frozen vegetables may be less likely to contain added sugar than canned. But READ THE LABEL. There are also numerous frozen vegetables that come in microwaveable steaming bags.

- Most mayonnaise today is laden with added sugar. **DUKE'S mayonnaise** is an excellent sugar free mayonnaise. There are a few others on the market, so ***read labels***.

- The fattiest cuts of meat and poultry are budgeted due entirely to the fat content. These foods are ***not*** bad for you and there is no other reason for the limitation.

- DO NOT eat the maximum portions allowed of every Budgeted Food item all the time. Use common sense, these items are allowed, but are meant to be eaten in moderation.

- Fruit juice should generally be avoided due to the high sugar content of these beverages. Grapefruit juice, Lemon juice and Lime juice are the only exceptions to this rule.

- TAKE VITAMINS. Take all the vitamins you want. Vitamins will never hurt you, and will help substantially. You will find more detailed information on vitamins later in this book.

- Fiber is very important for a variety of reasons. If you are NOT eating 25 to 30 grams of fiber a day, you may want to take a fiber supplement (Chia Seeds added to beverages are an EXCELLENT source of fiber and protein! Benefiber types of supplements are also good).

    - Solulable Fiber (found in apples, broccoli, etc.) forms a gel-like substance in the stomach and slows the movement of food, which makes you feel full longer. Solulable Fiber has also been shown to lower cholesterol.

    - INsolulable Fiber (found in celery, fresh greens, etc.) speeds the movement of food through the intestines which may prevent the absorption of calories. It also slows down the absorption of sugar, which is very good for those of us trying to manage our weight. Insolulable Fiber has also been shown to decrease the risk of some cancers due to the fact that it lowers the body's exposure to toxins.

- If you have a craving for a starch, a potato is the best carbohydrate of the starch world. When eaten, a potato feeds into your system slowly and completely. If you must eat a starch, eat a small potato.

- Corn is unique. Even though it is a starchy vegetable, your system does not break down whole kernel fresh corn. (If you don't believe me, just watch your toilet for it to come out after you have eaten it). Corn is a great source of fiber, too. Eat ***ONLY*** whole kernel corn with ***NO ADDED sugar***. A little salt or butter is fine. Frozen whole kernel corn can easily be microwaved.

- CARBOHYDRATES AND MANY ALCOHOLIC BEVERAGES CONVERT TO SUGAR during the digestive process. This is why both carbohydrates and alcohol are limited or forbidden on this program.

- Many of the Forbidden Beverages contain alcohol. I believe alcohol is fine, and in fact have already told you my #1 Essential Edible is wine, but not all alcoholic beverages are equal. The alcoholic beverages that are on the Forbidden Beverages list are there due to very high sugar content. It is best to avoid these particular beverages. Certainly at least avoid them until you have achieved your weight goal, and after that, drink them only very rarely.

- Starchy vegetables, such as eggplant, squash, pumpkin, lima beans and peas are also on the FORBIDDEN list due to the high starch and sugar content that will flood your system if eaten.

- You have probably noted that aside from half an English muffin with breakfast, bread is not allowed. Bread is generally an empty carbohydrate, and turns right into sugar in your system. In fact, I would recommend you skip the half English muffin at breakfast. But if you must have SOME bread, it is best to eat it in the morning, as you are much more likely to burn it off.

- Wraps are allowed in limited quantities, but you would be better off to avoid sandwiches when possible (if you are constantly on the go, or in meetings where lunches are ordered in without consulting the attendees, this may be a challenge). If you ***Must*** eat a sandwich, eat only half the bread (take off one slice of bread and eat carefully, or use a knife and fork). I eat cheeseburgers with NO bread, and put the mayonnaise on the side for dipping. Or if I MUST have a piece of bread, only 1 piece under the burger. DO NOT eat bread at night unless it is completely unavoidable.

- If you are on the go and the *ONLY* viable choice is a fast food sandwich, order something with protein in it. Turkey and cheese, a cheese burger, roast beef and cheese, with whatever condiment you like. EAT THE FILLING, toss the bread.

- A wrap is always a better choice than bread.

- If you are in a business meeting and lunch is brought in, choose a tuna salad or a chicken salad sandwich. Eat the filling with a fork and leave the bread on the plate. Eat a couple of pickles; skip the macaroni salad and potato chips. Don't even LOOK at the cookies and brownies.

- If you are in an early morning meeting, have coffee or tea. Skip the bagels and pastries. If you are ***starving*** and afraid you'll pass out, choose an apple if one is available OR have ¼ of a bagel with butter or cream cheese. But you SHOULD have had your breakfast long before you arrived at the meeting – I know, life happens, emergencies arise. We've all had those mornings where the dog ate the homework, the kids missed the bus, you had no choice but to throw on your clothes, take the kids to school and rush to your meeting . . . late. That's why ***Dynamic Dining Design*** allows all the flexibility, so life can happen and you can ***still*** work with the program.

- Protein Salads: Tuna Salad, Chicken Salad, Ham Salad, Turkey or Smoked Turkey Salad, Crab Salad (real crab), Lobster Salad – all of these are fantastic choices for your protein. ***However***, it is critical to insure there is NO added sugar, bread crumbs or fillers in the salad itself, in the mayonnaise used, or in any of the ingredients – especially if the salad is packaged or purchased at a deli. The following simple recipe makes an excellent protein salad:

    - Protein (Tuna, Chicken, Turkey, Shrimp, etc.)
    - Sugar Free Mayonnaise
    - Mustard (if desired)

  - Celery
  - Onion
  - Dill Pickle
  - Cucumber
  - Lemon Juice (optional)
  - Diced Egg (optional)
  - Salt (optional)
  - Vinegar (optional)

- AVOID COLD CUTS. Cold cuts are generally full of sugar and other additives that are not good for weight loss. I recommend you avoid them completely. But, if it is impossible to avoid cold cuts completely, definitely limit cold cuts to twice a week maximum.

- Many people do not realize what additives, fillers, processing and other alterations do to food. For instance – Canadian Bacon (with no added sugar, such as maple curing) is low calorie and has less than 1 carb per slice. Regular bacon has 4 to 10 carbs for every 2 slices, depending on brand and added sugar. Pepperoni, knockwurst and salami have less than 1 carb per ounce. Bologna and bratwurst have 5 to 12 carbs per ounce.

- Tuna salad, chicken salad, ham salad, turkey or smoked turkey salad, shrimp salad, crab salad (real crab that is), and lobster salad are all fantastic choices. HOWEVER, you must insure there is NO added sugar, bread crumbs or fillers in the salad itself, the mayonnaise used, or in any of the ingredients. See the appendixes at the end for an excellent protein salad recipe.

- Barbeque is forbidden because it is not only full of fat and should only be eaten very rarely under the best of circumstances, but it is also absolutely full of sugar and goodness knows what else!

- **DO NOT** indiscriminately add foods that are **NOT** on the lists just because you know the food you want to add is low calorie and low carb. Many foods were purposely eliminated from Dynamic Dining Design because they inhibit weight loss or chemically interact with other foods in ways that are detrimental to metabolism.

- **If you have a question about a specific food, please send an e-mail to the e-mail address at the end of the book.**

- **This last is a secret, *don't even tell yourself*.** Forbidden Foods aren't COMPLETELY forbidden forever. BUT you SHOULD AVOID THEM COMPLETELY until you achieve your weight goal and after that treat these foods as the forbidden treats they are. Once every 3 to 4 months for any Forbidden Food is more than plenty.

LET'S GET PHYSICAL!

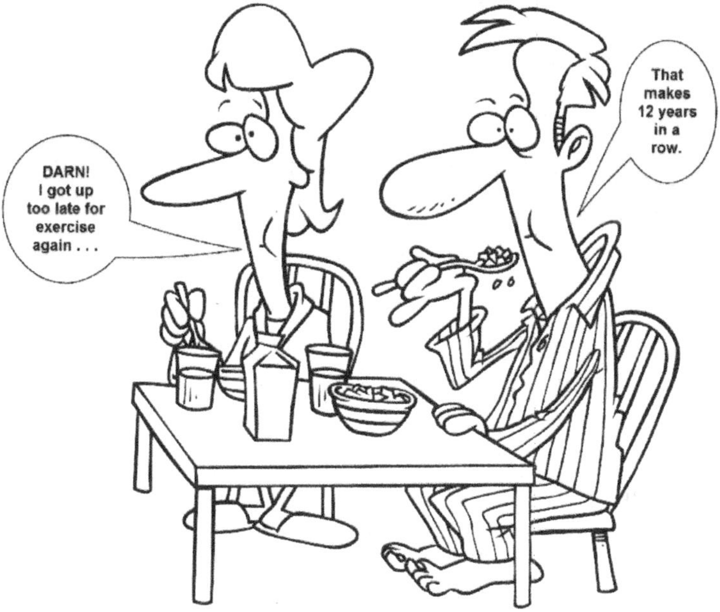

There is no way of sugar coating it, exercise is an absolute imperative. Can you lose weight without exercising? Possibly. If there were medical conditions preventing you from losing weight that have been resolved or are finally being effectively treated, it's even probable you will lose weight without exercising.

But, if you do not exercise, you won't be as healthy as you should be. No matter how attractive couch potatoland appears, and no matter how overweight and out of shape you are, some physical activity is a good thing. Exercise boosts your mood (yes it does), you sleep better, you look better, and it strengthens your immune system.

You don't have to go to the gym (you already know how I feel about that), and the activity (or activities) you choose shouldn't make you miserable. There is no need for marathon training or Olympic competition. BUT you must get your blood circulating a little faster, you need to get more oxygen into your system, and if possible, you need to get your heart rate up at least a few times a week. It's good for you!

I promise after a week or so you will start to feel more energetic and the exercise will get easier.

Remember, start at your own pace. If you can only do 5 minutes of exercise per day, 3 or 4 days a week, do 5 minutes. Increase your time to 7 minutes ***when YOU are ready***. Do **NOT** let anyone guilt you into increasing your time before you are ready. But never forget, the GOAL is to be doing 30 minutes of exercise 3 or 4 times a week eventually. Keep that goal in mind, and work toward it, regardless of how long it takes to reach that goal.

There is no reason for exercise to be painful or make you miserable. In fact, if your chosen activity results in either pain or misery, you've chosen badly. Why are you punishing yourself? Exercise can be fun if you choose an activity you actually enjoy.

You can join a group to pursue your activity, or you can do your chosen exercise at home with the shades drawn. It doesn't matter as long as you are up and moving.

This chapter contains a list of activities that you might choose from. Or choose something you love that is not on the list. As long as it is an activity that gets you moving and gets your heart rate up a little bit, that's all that matters.

If you are as overweight and out of shape as I was at 274 pounds, and your chosen exercise/activity is something that is moderately strenuous, you should absolutely have your doctor approve what you are doing, and certify that you are physically able to do it from a medical perspective.

If you don't want to check with your doctor before starting an exercise routine, WALKING is ALWAYS a good start. I've never heard of a doctor telling their patients not to walk.

Walking is something everyone can do, regardless of where you are or what time of day or night it is. If you are in a hotel in an unfamiliar city and it is the middle of the night, take the elevator to the floor where the conference rooms are (which is generally deserted late at night), and walk up and down the hallways for your allotted time.

So no excuses. If you need any equipment or paraphernalia for your chosen exercise activity, make sure you have what you need, and get started.

EXERCISE/ACTIVITY SUGGESTIONS

Walking — Around the block, around the park, around the hotel floor, around the back yard, or on a treadmill in front of the television. If doesn't matter how you do it, walking is great exercise. Take it at your own pace and enjoy!

Dancing — Always fun, always enjoyable. Dancing of any type gets you moving and gets your blood circulating. Join a class, or get one of those dance video games for gaming systems and dance in front of your TV, or just put on your walkman or your iPod and boogie down.

Swimming — Swimming is wonderful exercise. Even just walking in the water provides added resistance and makes the exercise even more fun. Whether you have your own pool, one of those "endless" lap pools (lucky you if you do), or you go to the local community pool; swimming or exercising in water is enjoyable and great for you.

Golf — Can be a great exercise, especially if you walk the course rather than riding in one of the electric golf carts. If you're not in great shape, take a caddy with you to carry those heavy clubs.

Skating — Whether its roller skating or ice skating, always great exercise, always fun.

Martial Arts —Excellent exercise, good discipline, and, if you choose the right class or teacher, good for the spirit as well.

Biking — Whether you're outdoors riding a bike, or you are in the gym or in front of your own TV on a stationary bike of some kind, it's great exercise.

Fencing — Is lots of fun and more exercise that you can imagine if you've never done it.

Horseback Riding — Of course you have to have a horse (or rent one) and a reasonably nearby place to do it, but if you have access, horseback riding is great exercise, and it's fun.

Tennis — of course this takes two, unless the court where you play has one of those machines that shoot balls at you. Squash or Racquetball are also good options.

HOME EXERCISE EQUIPMENT

There is a great deal of home exercise equipment that you can invest in if you want to, but many of the machines you can buy don't provide the kind of work-out that you need. Here are a few suggestions of machines that you could purchase and get the right kind of exercise:

- A Walking Desk – yep, you heard me. Look it up on the internet. There are several companies that make desks that essentially come with a (slow moving) treadmill and the desk stands at a height where you can work standing up. This is great if you work at home and can invest in one.
- A Stationary Bike – Numerous varieties are available.
- A Ski Machine – Numerous companies make these.
- An Orbital or Elliptical Machine – Hundreds of models are available.
- An Orbitron – If you have the space and the financial ability to make the investment, this is fantastic, zero impact, exercise.

GYM MEMBERSHIP

If you enjoy the social aspects and don't have the same hang-ups I do, this is an excellent option and should give you a variety of activities to choose from. If the gym you choose has a pool, even better.

TEAM SPORTS

Team Sports are generally more strenuous and, of course, require a team or two. But all are outstanding exercise, including: football, baseball, basketball, hockey, soccer, rugby, volleyball, racquet ball, handball, water polo, etc.

CALORIES BURNED DURING ACTIVITIES

It is not necessary to figure out how many calories you are burning during exercise. As I have said many times, the old calories in/calories out nonsense is just that – nonsense. In fact, I'm not even sure it's advisable to know how many calories you are burning, it may just discourage you! However, for those of you who are cursed with insatiable curiosity, below is a very simplistic overview of calories burned by the minute based upon your individual weight for some of the most basic activities.

Why based on your weight? Well, a person who weighs 120 pounds burns fewer calories by walking for 20 minutes than a person who weighs 200 pounds. It stands to reason, the 120 pound person is moving far less weight right?

So, for the activities listed below, multiply the number of calories burned per minute BY YOUR WEIGHT, and then multiply again by the number of minutes you exercise. For example, if you weigh 225 pounds and you walk at 2.5 mph for 30 minutes, the calculation would be:

0.029 calories x 225 lbs = 6.5 calories/min

6.5 calories x 30 minutes walking = 195 calories burned

CALORIES BURNED PER MINUTE

Lying down/sleeping	0.0087
Sitting	0.0120
Standing	0.0156
Walking 2.5 mph	0.0240
Walking 3.5 mph	0.0340
Golf (4some)	0.0280
Bicycling 5.5 mph	0.0240
Swimming ¼ mph	0.0340
Skating (roller)	0.0389
Skating (ice) 10 mph	0.0325
Fencing	0.0340
Horse Back Riding	0.0389
Tennis	0.0475
Dancing	0.0433

As I said before, this is not an important calculation. The point is to get your blood circulating, your lungs working and to increase your energy. The benefit of exercise (even a little exercise) far exceeds the pathetic number of calories burned while you actually ARE exercising.

DESIGN BY MOTHER NATURE

Approximately 35 million years ago a population of tree climbing primates called *Aegyptopithecus* became the distant ancestor of the first hominid. It took about 20 Million years for evolution to slowly gestate that first hominid from the ancestral primates. So the very earliest hominid appeared on the scene some 15 Million years ago.

Fast forward another 14,800,000 evolutionary years and a pinnacle of evolutionary achievement was achieved when early modern man finally appeared on the Earth a short 200,000 years ago.

Our bodies operate pretty much the way nature intended them to be based on 15 million years of human evolutionary history.

It is important to be aware of how very slowly and selectively evolution (and any substantive changes in the way our bodies operate) actually occurs. In evolutionary terms, 100 years is about a nanosecond.

If you think about it, it is not really surprising that over 68% percent of the population is overweight. After all, it was not until the last 50 years or so (since sometime in the 1960s) that durable sources of sufficient available food have been dependable and the majority of the Earth's population has actually gotten enough (or more than enough) to eat on a regular basis.

Even as recently as the early 1900s only wealthy people really got enough (or too much) to eat on a continuous basis. A high percentage of the world population faced hunger, starvation or outright famine on a regular basis, even here in the United States. In fact, I have read that Audrey Hepburn's gamine figure was a direct result of the near starvation conditions she endured growing up in London during World War II.

Before 1900 erratic food supply problems were much worse and daily hunger, starvation, or famine situations were quite common worldwide.

As a result of the unpredictable availability of food faced by our ancestors during 99.999% of the last 15 Million years, nature designed our bodies to adjust quickly to sudden changes in the available supply of food. In times of plenty our bodies immediately build up stores of fat to protect against times of deprivation. In times of deprivation our bodies instantly adjust to burn fewer calories and relentlessly retain fat so that our bodies and our species will endure. It's probably going to take ***ANOTHER*** 15 or 20 Million years of evolution before nature catches up with the concept of 24 x 7 worldwide availability of Big Macs and Supersized Fries.

With this background in mind, it's easier to understand why it's so important for everyone, especially those of us with metabolism problems, to eat fairly consistently, and not make sudden dramatic changes in the amount and type of food we consume.

Our bodies are hardwired by nature to interpret a disruption in the amount of food we normally consume (such as one of those temporary things known as a "diet") to be a starvation situation. Going on a "diet" causes your body to immediately marshal its forces and adjust your metabolism to rigorously conserve fuel (tenaciously preserving your FAT). This is why one of the side effects of dieting is fatigue; your body is valiantly attempting to force you to ***do less*** so you burn less fat. THEN, when you go OFF the "diet" (there's that ugly word again) and revert to eating "normally" (i.e., more), your body happily interprets this as a "good harvest" situation, and adjusts to store fat as quickly as it can in anticipation of the next "famine".

This is why when we go on a "diet" (temporarily eating less) and then go off it (back to eating "normally," or more), so many of us immediately gain back the weight we lost PLUS a few extra pounds that have come along to the party with their friends to punish us for trying to evict them in the first place. This is why "Yo-Yo" dieters end up weighing more than when they started out.

Our bodies are designed by nature to vigorously defy all our efforts to lose weight, especially if we take temporary measures and make sudden drastic changes in our eating habits (i.e. go on a "diet"). Consequently, it is critical to strategize, and fool our body into complacency so it **doesn't notice** that we're downsizing. Thus, ***Dynamic Dining Design***, your new lifetime weight management strategy.

I am sure every woman in the world has noticed it seems to be easier for men to lose weight that it is for women to lose weight. It's true, it **IS** easier for men to lose weight – it's a scientific fact. Want to know why? Once again, it's the way pesky old Mother Nature designed us. We already know that women are smarter than men, but nature also decided men aren't as critical to the perpetuation of the species as women. In a famine situation, men's bodies are designed to last 3 months before they die; women's bodies with greater fat storage capability (which gives us our curves and feminine figures) and our body's far greater tenacity in preserving stores of fat, are designed to last 9 MONTHS before we die. This way pregnant females will have time to give birth so the species is guaranteed to propagate and a baby will be born before the poor woman finally dropped dead of starvation. Neat, isn't it?

And the current effect of this elegant innovation of nature, which insured the perpetuation of the human species, is that women gain weight easier and have a heck of a harder time losing it in this brave new world of plenty of supersized fast-food.

Now you hopefully understand why it is important to eat consistently and on a schedule to the best of your ability. Eating both meals and snacks on a reasonable schedule will insure you never get overly hungry. This way your body adjusts to your new eating habits without going into "starvation" mode. Over the long term making gradual changes to your Dining habits will help your body regulate your weight more consistently. Always remember that sudden dramatic changes or inconsistent eating habits result in greater production and more tenacious storage of fat.

It is equally important to exercise at ***RANDOM*** times (if possible), so your cagey body doesn't have a chance to stage a coup d'état and adjust to regularly scheduled exercise, by burning fewer calories at the time of day you normally engage in exercise. Yes, it's true. If you exercise on a regular schedule, scientific studies have shown your body will adjust to burn fewer calories at the time of day you have regularly scheduled for exercise.

To add to the madness, today there are many foods readily available to us that nature never anticipated.

For instance, refined sugar has only been around for a few hundred years, since the middle ages. Before that, if a food was sweetened, it was sweetened primarily with honey, or with fruit. Our body absorbs and processes honey or even fruit very differently than it handles refined sugar. What's more, sugar is more addictive than heroin.

Today refined sugar is added to virtually everything we eat. Sometimes you won't even recognized that sugar is in your food when you read the nutritional label, because food manufacturers have cleverly disguised the word "sugar" to sound like some harmless chemical, thus increasing our weight and addicting us to their product at the same time!

It is not just what we eat, most of the conditions in which we live have also changed dramatically in the past 50 to 100 years. Prior to 1950 air conditioning didn't exist. Before 1965 air conditioning was not common in most residential homes. Today virtually everyone lives and works in air conditioned bliss.

I have read theories that since our bodies burn more energy to keep us warm when we are cold, you should turn down your air conditioning and keep your environment's temperature uncomfortably cold to help you lose weight. HOWEVER, doing this could have the opposite effect – in a winter situation our bodies are designed to adjust to the change in temperature by storing ***more fat*** to keep us warm. So keeping your environment cold could cause you to gain weight.

One diet guru posited that raising the temperature of your environment until you are uncomfortably ***warm*** will trigger your body to shed weight.

I don't know which is right, and it could be that one method will work for some people and the opposite will work for others. I personally don't believe room temperature will play a big role in weight management for most of us. But if one method or the other actually does have an effect on your weight, by all means use it to your advantage.

The way we live and work and use our leisure time and eat is dramatically different today than at any previous time in human history. But to lose weight successfully and permanently it is imperative to understand how evolution designed our bodies.

It's a little like playing chess – I'm not a chess player myself, but I've always been told that a good chess player knows the next several moves they plan to make based on how they ***know*** their opponent will move in response.

In planning for permanent weight loss, strategy is everything and it's important to recognize that your body is your opponent. In order to plan a strategy that will achieve a successful result, it is crucial to understand what tactics your body is going to utilize to retaliate and attempt to foil your plans.

The only path to success involves a stealth strategy so your body remains complacent and doesn't realize downsizing is under way.

The point of the information in this chapter is to help you understand how your body has been designed to work – at least until evolution catches up with current conditions, which won't happen in our lifetime! Now you can see why the Dynamic Dining Design program is a strategy that will result in restructuring your body to the correct size and help insure you are winning the battle with your body.

Of course, there is ALSO ***supposed to be*** a natural weight regulator that helps your body keep your weight at an optimum setting that is not too heavy and not too thin. Those "magic genes" that some people have in abundant supply. The

Magic Factor that has apparently failed to operate properly in the rest of us.

In the next sections of this book you will find information that will help you figure out what health problems may be negatively affecting your ability to lose weight and find a doctor to diagnose and treat those issues. Solving any health issues that are impacting your ability to lose weight combined with the Dynamic Dining Design way of life should cause your internal systems to re-set your body's natural ability to properly regulate your weight and activate your own "Magic" Factor!

WHEN PIGS FLY!

I'll bet no one has ever bothered to tell you, it's ***impossible*** to lose weight if you have certain medical issues, pigs will fly first. But, treat the problem and voila! Suddenly you're downsizing.

It was difficult to decide which issues to tackle first in this section. Each type of health condition deserves its own chapter. But many of the health problems plaguing people who are overweight are interrelated and it's sort of a chicken or egg type of question – which comes first?

At the end of September 2010, I was morbidly obese. I had lifelong thyroid and metabolism problems, I had Type 2 Diabetes, high cholesterol, high tri-glycerides, very high C-Reactive Protein (that no medical professional had been able to explain for years), was at high risk for a heart attack or stroke, had joint pain in my ankles and knees so bad I could barely walk sometimes, acid reflux, and – oh yeah – I had ***just*** been diagnosed with Obstructive Sleep Apnea so severe it could have been fatal.

Since my newest internist had, in June of 2010, changed my thyroid medication to Armour Thyroid, and his colleague who was now my endocrinologist/weight loss specialist had, about the same time, insisted I start taking phentermine – explaining it did not ***just*** control appetite (which I didn't need), it ***ALSO*** increased your metabolism (which I desperately needed), I had lost 3 pounds over the course of 4 months bringing my weight to 281 by mid-September.

It was the first three pounds I had lost in about 12 years and I was grateful. But by my calculation, it would take me about 13.5 years to lose the additional 140 pounds or so I still needed to lose!

It came as a tremendous surprise to me when I suddenly lost 4 pounds during the last two weeks of September. Could the new medications have suddenly kicked my body into overdrive? I certainly wasn't eating any differently. So I was happy to be down the additional 4 pounds, but I didn't understand it. At that point for me to lose 4 pounds in two weeks seemed miraculous!

So, there I was sitting in the office of the doctor who had ordered the sleep study that resulted in the Sleep Apnea diagnosis. Looking over my chart, he casually asked me how I was doing with my new CPAP machine, and he congratulated me on losing the 4 pounds.

I told him the CPAP machine was fine, I was sleeping like a baby through the entire night. But confessed I was surprised to have lost 4 pounds so quickly because I wasn't doing anything differently from the prior months I'd been seeing him.

He said, "Sure you are, the CPAP machine is letting you sleep; probably for the first time in years."

I said yes, that was nice, but that wouldn't cause me to lose that much weight that fast.

He looked up from my chart and very matter of factly said, "Of course it did. It's impossible to lose weight if you have sleep apnea." And he looked back at my chart, as if he hadn't just said something earth-shattering.

Those were the most galvanizing words I had ever heard. They had the ring of a clarion bell to me. Me, the person who had spent 110% of the last 35 years learning everything possible and doing everything possible relative to weight loss and weight management. And the doctor acted as if this were an insignificant fact I should have somehow known!

If he dropped a bomb in the room it couldn't have had a more dramatic effect on me. I was simply stunned, overwhelmed, breath taken; there aren't words to even begin to describe how I felt. I couldn't speak or even formulate an intelligent question.

WHAT!!!!!! THEN WHY DIDN'T ANY OF THE OVERPRICED, SUPPOSEDLY BRILLIANT, WEIGHT-LOSS/METABOLISM SPECIALISTS I'D BEEN SEEING FOR TWO DECADES EVER SAY THIS TO ME BEFORE? WOULD IT HAVE BEEN SO HARD TO SUGGEST I MIGHT BE A VICTIM OF SLEEP APNEA????? ***Why didn't anybody at least ever check???***

Sure, a couple of doctors along the way had asked if I had ever been ***DIAGNOSED*** with sleep apnea, but when the response from me was "No," they checked off a box and moved on to the next question.

I had read hundreds of books on the subject of weight loss, and a few of them had mentioned that if you don't get sufficient sleep it will make losing weight more difficult. But *NONE* of the books said much more than that about it. One sentence in 300 pages hardly raises sleep to a critical level.

NOT ONE DOCTOR I HAD EVER TALKED TO had ever so much as *HINTED* that sleep apnea or other sleep disorders could be a systemic cause or the root problem related to my inability to lose weight for the past decade or two!!!!! Even this doctor had only off-handedly decided a sleep study would be a good idea to "rule out" sleep apnea as a factor.

WHY, IN THE NAME OF ALL THAT'S HOLY, had no one ever said this was a *CRITICAL* factor??? What if I had said no to the Sleep Study, due to financial or other factors? Would this doctor have simply moved on without ever saying anything more? The scary thing is, he probably **would** have just checked a box and moved on.

Still in shock, I actually got through the few remaining minutes of the appointment, politely thanking the doctor, who told me he was looking forward to my visit the next month to see how much weight I had lost by then.

I took my prescriptions from him and checked out in the lobby, even managing to make polite small talk with the receptionist as she waited for the credit card charge to go through. Miraculously, I made it into a cab and headed home. Even after arriving home I had *STILL* not actually processed the bombshell this doctor had dropped on me.

When I got home I sat down and had a couple of glasses of wine to help me find some calm in my internal storm. I talked to my husband about what the doctor had told me. By that time I had a better grip on myself, but I was still in turmoil, and now I realized I was angry.

I had always had metabolism problems and, from the first time a doctor finally admitted I might have a thyroid problem in 1979 to the spring of 2010, I had generally had to educate myself and suggest to the doctors – even the high priced specialists – what tests should be run and what medications "we" might think about trying. Prior to today's robust internet information highway, this was a much more difficult, time consuming task than it is today. And even today it isn't easy, because there is SO MUCH doctors either **don't even know** or **won't** tell you. And even with books, research materials and the internet available, there is still so much mis-information, and such huge gaps in the information that exists, it is still a nearly impossible chore!

BUT SLEEPING! I have had problems sleeping since . . . well, forever. Some of my earliest memories have to do with being unable to fall asleep. My parents always talked about what a night owl I was, even when I was just two or three years old. But when I was young, my sleep problems revolved primarily around actually FALLING asleep. Once I got into my thirties my sleep problems had morphed, and I was waking up around 4:00 am and couldn't go back to sleep easily, so I got up tired or exhausted in the mornings.

By age 40 I was having such bad night sweats that I would wake up soaking wet in a puddle in the bed in the middle of the night. I frequently joked that I was having the longest peri-menopause in the history of woman! I gained weight continuously, no matter what I did, no matter what I did or did not eat, nothing, **nothing**, ***nothing*** would stop the pounds from attaching themselves to my body!! And no doctor had ***EVER ONCE*** suggested I might have sleep apnea.

I had my first sleep study ***EVER*** on September 15th, 2010 only because this doctor had told me that it would be a good idea to do it just to "***rule out***" everything he could think of that might be affecting my ability to lose weight.

The night of the actual sleep study, I finally managed to fall asleep in spite of the numerous wires and electrodes attached to me. I had no sooner fallen asleep than the staff woke me up to put a CPAP machine on me. In the morning I found out the Medical Director of the Weill Cornell Sleep Center came in on an emergency basis especially to see me. I was told I had such ***severe Obstructive Sleep Apnea*** that the medical technicians monitoring my sleep woke her in the middle of the night because my blood oxygen levels fell to 44% shortly after I fell asleep. This was such a critical and dangerous situation that she had ordered the technicians to immediately hook me up to a CPAP machine, rather than continuing the study without it. She told me it was likely that I had been suffering from ever worsening sleep apnea for at least a decade, and probably even longer.

A CPAP machine was delivered to my house on an emergency basis at the behest of the doctor. From the first night using the CPAP I slept like a baby. Amazingly, those first 4 pounds were just the tip of the iceberg. As soon as I started sleeping every night with the CPAP machine (since by that time I was already ***finally*** on the correct thyroid medication, Armour Thyroid, and the phentermine to boost my sluggish metabolism) weight began to literally fall off!

A decade or more of Sleep Apnea (I now actually believe at least 15 years of undiagnosed sleep apnea) definitely correlated with the period of time in my life during which "difficult to lose weight" became "impossible to lose weight." So what the doctor had said to me began to make more sense in light of the difficulties I had been experiencing over the prior twelve to fifteen years.

As soon as I was able to breathe again, I got on the internet and started searching. Varying sites gave varying lists of symptoms AND wildly varying lists of the EFFECTS caused by Sleep Apnea AND the concomitant sleep deprivation that goes along with it.

Who knew??!! I had no idea. And, even reading every bit of current research on the subject while armed with my new found knowledge, nowhere did I find the information I was searching for. I found hundreds of studies and web pages on Sleep Apnea that say one of the symptoms may be weight gain. BUT, there are literally hundreds of conditions that list possible weight gain as a symptom.

NO WHERE up to now, has anyone posted a sign in HUGE neon letters that says

IF YOU HAVE SLEEP APNEA it will be LITERALLY IMPOSSIBLE for you to LOSE WEIGHT *UNTIL* you get TREATEMENT!!

It quickly became very clear to me that the sleep disorders, combined with my metabolism problems, had caused the perfect storm and had resulted in the weight problems I had been living with for the past several decades at least – maybe my entire life!!!

It began to dawn on me how vastly irresponsible all the doctors I had seen over the past two or three decades had been. Numerous, supposedly brilliant, doctors (some of whose names have been mentioned in national publications) to whom I had paid literally tens of thousands of dollars.

What else hadn't they told me??!! I intended to find out!

THE LAND OF NOD
(Ah … For A Good Night's Sleep)

If you cannot lose weight (or if you lose an unreasonably small amount of weight) regardless of what you eat or what you do, ***RUN***, do not walk, ***TO THE NEAREST SLEEP DISORDER SPECIALIST***. Tell the specialist whatever you need to tell them to compel them to order a sleep study for you. ***DO NOT*** tell them you can't lose weight, this will (sadly) probably be meaningless to a doctor who specializes in sleep disorders.

Even though there are many types of sleep disorders, my suggestion is that you tell the specialist you believe you have sleep apnea, and describe to them some of the list of symptoms in this chapter, keep adding additional symptoms to your list until they agree to order a sleep study for you. Due to all the attention sleep apnea has received the last few years, it is the easiest thing you can tell a doctor that will result in a sleep study being ordered.

The first priority is to ***GET*** the sleep study ordered. If you have a sleep disorder (any sleep disorder), a sleep study should result in a diagnosis and even if more tests are necessary the study will, at the very least, identify the fact that you have a problem which needs to be diagnosed and treated.

If you are convincing, the doctor ***SHOULD*** provide a diagnosis of a suspected sleep disorder, and your insurance ***SHOULD*** pay for both the doctor visit and the sleep study.

Depending on the type of medical insurance you have, you may have to go through a primary care physician in order to get an appointment with a Sleep Specialist.

BE AWARE that if your insurance company requires that you go to your primary care physician ***BEFORE*** you can see a specialist, it is highly likely that the primary care physician is actually being **paid bonuses** by the insurance company to *DISALLOW AND DISCOURAGE* the use of specialists. In this type of scenario the primary care physician (who is there primarily to vigorously guard and defend the gate between you and actual decent medical care) will have a hundred reasons why you ***DON'T NEED*** to see a Sleep Specialist.

INSIST that you and your significant other with whom you are sleeping are *CERTAIN* that you have sleep apnea. *DO NOT* allow the primary care physician to simply prescribe sleeping pills and send you home. Keep expanding the list of symptoms and side effects you are suffering until the primary care physician has no other choice than to refer you to a Sleep Specialist.

Although there are more than 70 documented sleep disorders; the most common sleep disorders include Sleep Apnea, Insomnia, Restless Leg Syndrome, and Narcolepsy. It is estimated that there are more than 20 million people suffering from undiagnosed, untreated sleep disorders. I personally believe that estimate is very low.

This chapter provides an overview of sleep disorders, how sleep (or lack thereof) affects your weight, and the crippling effects sleep deprivation and sleep disorders can have on your body's ability to regulate your weight normally.

It is highly likely you will learn things from this chapter you have never known before. That is what this book is about, giving you information, and/or presenting information that may be available but was presented in such a way that it seemed unimportant in terms of weight loss or weight management. Information is power, and this book will empower you by presenting information in ways you have never seen it presented or interpreted before – making the information meaningful and understandable in relation to your weight.

I am concerned specifically with what you need to know in order to achieve weight loss and normal weight regulation – empowering you so you can finally achieve activation of your very own, god given, "magic genes"!

Since I have no intention of writing a scientific treatise (and why would you want to read one?) I am not highly focused on providing scads of scientific sources or reference materials, although there are a few references of some of the most important issues in the Reference section of this book. If you want additional information or more detailed information, there are so many scientific papers and so much information available on sleep studies and sleep disorders you will probably have difficulty finding the time to read them all! (For links to some of these information sources, please visit our web site.) But very few of the information sources or studies on sleep disorders actually discuss how these conditions affect your weight management in any detail.

Some sources indicate that sleep is important if you want to lose weight. The most dramatic statement I have seen says something like: "*It is important to make sure you are getting good night's sleep if you are trying to lose weight. Research has shown that on average individuals who do not get sufficient sleep are heavier than those who do. Scientists now believe there may be a link between obesity and lack of sleep.*"

The *ONE* statement you will *NOT FIND ANYWHERE* is this:

IF you are NOT getting adequate, high quality sleep on a regular basis, you WILL GAIN WEIGHT, AND you will find it IMPOSSIBLE to lose weight!

If you have a sleep disorder, first of all you may not even ***know*** that you do. Second, it is a foregone conclusion you are not experiencing a natural, normal sleep cycle (getting a good night's sleep) *ANY* night. Third, you are sleep deprived. Consequently you will find it impossible to lose weight!! The most common sleep disorders are:

- Sleep Apnea
- Insomnia
- Restless Leg Syndrome
- Narcolepsy

SLEEP DEPRIVATION

Most people do not realize how devastating sleep deprivation can be. While we are asleep, our bodies are very busy, repairing, reinvigorating and resetting physical and mental processes in our bodies and our brains. Sleep is restorative and keeps us young by slowing the aging process. While we sleep memory is consolidated, stored and appropriately filed for later access. If you don't sleep well, the most affected organ is your brain.

The simplest everyday things that we don't give a second thought to can disrupt sleep and impair the quality of our sleep – such as heartburn, bad dreams, physical discomfort, pain, noise, light, temperature or disruptive bed partners. Constant disruptions, even noise outside, or a light outside our window, anything that filters through to our sub-conscious, regardless of whether we remember actively waking, can result in sleep deprivation.

If you have a problem sleeping only 2 or 3 nights a week, whether it's trouble falling asleep, waking up during the night, waking up early and not being able to go back to sleep, or even just getting up in the morning feeling tired and unrefreshed, you may be sleep deprived and not even know it. Daytime sleepiness is a warning signal that you are ***NOT*** getting enough sleep. If you have daytime sleepiness, even infrequently, and you believe you are getting adequate sleep, it may be a symptom of a sleep disorder.

EFFECTS OF SHORT TERM SLEEP DEPRIVATION
(include, but are not limited to)

- Motor Vehicle Accidents (approximately 100,000 motor vehicle accidents each year are the result of sleep deprivation. Over 1,500 deaths result from these accidents)
- Accidents operating Machinery or Equipment
- Irritability
- Impatience
- Results in changes to the brain that cause cravings for high-calorie/high-carbohydrate comfort foods AND decreased will-power
- Decreased Productivity
- Poor Performance at Work
- Risk of Injury
- Safety Issues

EFFECTS OF LONG TERM SLEEP DEPRIVATION
(include, but are not limited to)

- **OBESITY**
- **INCREASED APPETITE**
- Serious Health Risks
- Serious Safety Risks

- Hyperglycemia
- Diabetes Type 2 (If you don't sleep 7 to 8 hours a night your risk of developing Type 2 Diabetes increases by a stunning 37% TO 88% according to recent studies.)
- Impaired ability of your body to utilize insulin
- Insulin resistance
- Low insulin production
- Difficulty exercising or lack of motivation to exercise
- Inability to complete tasks
- Job Loss
- High Blood Pressure
- Hypertension
- Cardiovascular Problems
- Cardiovascular Disease
- Inability to concentrate
- Impaired judgment
- Impaired decision making skills
- Impaired reasoning skills
- Seriously impaired mental processes
- Impaired Brain Function
- Negative Moods

- Depression
- Negative Behavior
- Impaired Social Skills
- Risk of Substance Abuse
- Impaired short term memory
- Early onset dementia
- Engaging in unsafe actions
- Accelerated Aging Process

SLEEP APNEA

In the most basic laymen's terms, sleep apnea is a condition wherein the individual repeatedly stops breathing during sleep. This results in frequent awakenings (20 to 30 per hour normally, although as many as 200+ awakenings per hour have been documented in very severe cases, however the sleeper generally ***DOES NOT KNOW*** they have awakened). Sleep apnea not only makes it impossible for a victim to lose weight, it is a dangerous, life threatening condition all on its own.

There is more than one type of sleep apnea, although it doesn't matter which type you have, the result will be the same: abnormal sleep patterns, sleep deprivation, oxygen starvation and a virtual *COMPLETE INABILITY to LOSE WEIGHT.*

Fortunately for nearly everyone who suffers from sleep apnea, the treatment is easy – use a CPAP or a Bi-PAP machine every night, as recommended by your doctor. You will quickly reverse most or all of the side effects of sleep apnea. ***AND you will virtually certainly INSTANTLY START LOSING WEIGHT***, possibly even dramatically.

SYMPTOMS OF SLEEP APNEA INCLUDE
(but are not limited to)

- Waking up numerous times during the night (most people who have sleep apnea don't even realize they are waking up, because the awakening is so brief, or the arousal doesn't fully awaken you, but it does disrupt your sleep)
- Snoring
- Gulping in your sleep
- Making noises in your sleep (other than talking)
- Abrupt awakening with shortness of breath
- Awakening with dry mouth or throat
- Difficulty staying asleep
- Fragmented sleep
- Exhaustion when you get up in the morning
- Daytime sleepiness
- Chronic Fatigue
- Morning Headaches

- Night sweats
- Low Blood Pressure
- Low blood oxygen
- Heart Palpitations or Heart Rhythm Abnormalities
- High C-Reactive Protein

SIDE EFFECTS OF SLEEP APNEA INCLUDE
(but are not limited to)

- **INABILITY TO LOSE WEIGHT**
- **OBESITY**
- Sleep deprivation
- Impaired ability to concentrate or focus attention
- Headaches
- Irritability
- Anxiety
- Depression
- Anger
- Short Term Memory Loss
- Impaired learning ability and executive function
- Mental confusion
- "Foggy" thinking

- Compromised judgmental reasoning
- Alteration in mood or chronic mood swings
- Depression
- Altered personality
- Impaired ability to drive or operate machinery
- Impaired motor abilities
- Increased risk of auto accident
- Impaired Reaction Time
- Poor job performance
- Loss of job
- Frequent urge to urinate at night
- Diabetes Type 2
- Impaired or compromised motivation to engage in physical activity or exercise
- Loss of balance
- Loss of coordination
- High cholesterol
- High triglycerides
- Acid Reflux
- High blood pressure
- Fast pulse
- Heart arrhythmia or abnormal heart rhythm

- Congestive heart failure
- Heart attack
- Stroke
- Decrease in quality of life
- **Most severely affected organ is the brain**
- Death
- Sleep apnea becomes more dangerous over time and is considered a federal Social Security disability

INSOMNIA

If you suffer from insomnia you are likely to be well aware of your condition. If you are not already under the care of a Sleep Specialist, you should find one immediately and get treatment.

Insomnia is fairly easy to understand. It is characterized by difficulty falling asleep and/or waking up in the night and having difficulty going back to sleep. The result is sleep deprivation AND **a compromised ability to lose weight OR AN INABILITY TO LOSE WEIGHT.**

Insomnia may be long term or short term and causal factors can include numerous things such as: emotional or physical disorders, stress, environmental noise, extreme temperatures, medication (prescription or non-prescription), and many other things. What many doctors won't tell you, OR don't even know, is that insomnia can be caused by Thyroid disorders. (See the chapter on thyroid disorders for more information.)

Unfortunately for sufferers of insomnia, discovering the root cause(s) of insomnia can be difficult. Generally, the treatment for insomnia is either to cure or correct the root cause so that the patient returns to a normal sleep pattern, OR (much more likely) to prescribe sleeping pills.

Sleeping pills are far from a perfect solution. Because science has not yet identified the specific combination of chemicals or hormones produced by our bodies that produce a natural sleep cycle, there is ***NO*** currently available sleeping pill that replicates an actual normal, natural night's sleep.

Having said this, taking sleeping pills is still preferable to not sleeping, and should result in weight loss if insomnia is your **only** problem.

SYMPTOMS OF INSOMNIA INCLUDE
(but are not limited to)

- Difficulty falling asleep
- Waking up in the night and having difficulty going back to sleep

SIDE EFFECTS OF INSOMNIA INCLUDE
(but are not limited to)

- Sleep deprivation
- Exhaustion upon waking up
- Daytime sleepiness

- *COMPROMISED ABILITY OR INABILITY TO LOSE WEIGHT*
- "Foggy" thinking
- Depression
- Mood swings

RESTLESS LEG SYNDROME

Restless leg syndrome is a condition that is usually chronic, and affects sufferers both when waking and when sleeping. In simple terms, restless leg syndrome is a neurologic disorder that causes burning and other unpleasant sensations in the legs, and causes its victims to have an overwhelming and irresistible urge to move their legs or to get up and walk around. Symptoms become worse during periods of inactivity, including sleep, which frequently results in disrupted sleep.

Treatments for restless leg syndrome range from exercise and massage in mild cases, to prescription medication for the worst cases. But in the most severe cases there are few medications that work well or continuously and most suffers of bad or severe restless leg syndrome suffer from sleep deprivation **AND a compromised ability to lose weight OR THE INABILITY TO LOSE WEIGHT**.

SYMPTOMS OF RESTLESS LEG INCLUDE
(but are not limited to)

- Burning or unpleasant sensations in the legs, especially when inactive or sleeping
- Overwhelming, irresistible urge to move legs or to get up and walk around

SIDE EFFECTS OF RESTLESS LEG INCLUDE
(but are not limited to)

- Sleep deprivation
- Exhaustion upon waking
- Daytime sleepiness
- **Compromised ability OR INABILITY TO LOSE WEIGHT**

NARCOLEPSY

Narcolepsy is a chronic disorder that affects several hundred thousand people in the U.S. alone, although it is estimated that less than half have been diagnosed. In the simplest terms, narcolepsy is excessive and overwhelming daytime sleepiness (even after an adequate amount of sleep). People with narcolepsy frequently have abnormal sleep cycles which may be the root cause of this terrible affliction, although the condition is not fully understood by science.

SYMPTOMS OF NARCOLEPSY INCLUDE
(but are not limited to)

- Overwhelming, irresistible daytime sleepiness
- Falling asleep suddenly during active waking hours
- Fragmented sleep
- Abnormal sleep patterns
- Hallucinations
- Cataplexy (muscle collapse without warning when awake)
- Sleep paralysis (temporary inability to talk or move when falling asleep or waking up)

SIDE EFFECTS OF NARCOLEPSY INCLUDE
(but are not limited to)

- Possible sleep deprivation
- Chronic Fatigue
- Depression
- **Compromised ability or INABILITY TO LOSE WEIGHT**

TO SLEEP, PERCHANCE TO DREAM

Sleep is like the ocean. As much as is known about sleep, there is much more that is unknown and the depths of sleep present an enormous number of mysteries to medical science. Almost everything that **IS** known about sleep has been learned in the last three decades. What **IS** known about sleep and circadian rhythms is fascinating, and what is **NOT** known is even more fascinating. I will do my best to keep this section as strictly as possible to how sleep affects your weight – which is ***DRAMATICALLY!!!*** Read on.

Sleep is ***NOT*** a period when our brain or our body shuts down so we can rest.

Most of the sleep cycle is a time when our brain and many parts of our bodies are even more active than when we are awake, we simply are not aware of what is happening!

There are five stages of sleep. All mammals and birds experience the same five stages, including REM sleep. However, the amount of the time spent sleeping during each 24 hour period, and the amount of time each stage of sleep lasts varies significantly from mammal to mammal. Scientists have no hard evidence that mammals other than humans dream. However, I defy anyone who has ever lived with an animal, whether a dog or a cat or a horse or a gerbil, to tell me that animals don't dream too.

It is unclear whether the lack of sleep causes weight gain, or whether lack of sleep keeps our metabolism from functioning properly, however it is crystal clear to me at this point that lack of high quality sleep will result in weight gain and an inability to lose weight.

There is also NO evidence that lack of sufficient, high quality sleep can cause overeating which will lead to weight gain. I am making the assumption that most of the people reading this book, like me, do not usually actually overeat. **IF** you are an overeater, for Pete's sake **STOP!** If you cannot stop on your own, you should have already followed my earlier advice. See virtually any doctor and get some diet pills. THEN follow the Dynamic Dining Design program. You will lose weight on the Dynamic Dining Design program if overeating is your only problem.

When we sleep our body disengages from the waking world in an active process where sensory perception is suppressed or blocked by our body. This blockage is milder in early stages of sleep, growing stronger as sleep progresses to the point that a state of perceptual blindness occurs during which we truly do not see visual stimuli in our environment. This is true even of people who sleep with their eyes open (rare and somewhat disconcerting phenomena. Auditory responses and responses to touch are similarly dampened to a very significant degree.

In a normal sleep cycle, there are 5 stages of sleep. What is now known as NREM (or Non-REM) sleep encompasses the first 4 stages.

- In Stage 1, alpha waves evolve into Theta waves as drowsiness resolves into actual sleep.

- In Stage 2, sleep becomes deeper and you become disengaged from your surroundings. Your breathing and heart rate remain regular, but your body temperature AND your brain temperature decreases. Sleeping in a cool room (which assists in this cooling process) can be helpful in falling asleep.

- In Stage 3 and Stage 4, the deepest Delta Wave sleep occurs. Brain activity decreases, your blood pressure drops, your breathing becomes slower, muscles relax, blood supply to muscles increases and a plethora of hormones and biochemicals are released.

- In Stage 5, the now famous REM (or Rapid Eye Movement) sleep, dramatic changes occur. Dreams unfurl. Brain activity increases in motor and sensory areas, but your body becomes almost immobile as our brain turns our muscles off so we don't act out our dreams. Usually movement during this stage is limited to muscle twitches primarily in fingers, toes and facial muscles as you respond to your dreams. Heart rate increases, blood pressure increases up to 30 percent, and breathing increases. Body temperature tends to vary based on room temperature. Cerebral blood flow increases dramatically by as much as 50% to 200% higher than waking levels. Eyes dart back and forth in rapid movements.

The 4 stages of NREM sleep last approximately 80 minutes, followed by an approximate 10 minute period of REM sleep. This 90 minute cycle repeats 3 to 6 times during the night. With each successive cycle the length of time occupied by Stage 3 and 4 Delta sleep decreases, and REM sleep increases somewhat.

Numerous concurrent events take place during a normal night's sleep. Fascinating physiological changes occur during NREM and REM sleep, as described above. But even more importantly, our bodies release chemicals and hormones most of which are primarily released ***OR are ONLY*** released when we sleep.

- Human Growth Hormone (HGH) is only released during sleep, generally during the early stages of sleep, and is tied to both sleep and circadian rhythm.
- Melatonin, a hormone produced by the pineal gland, is critical to both sleep and body repair processes. Melatonin has been associated with reversing certain types of cancer, and in a recent (2010) study where a breast tumor was bathed in Melatonin, the tumor reversed itself. Melatonin release is controlled completely by circadian rhythm and **Melatonin is *ONLY* released in the dark**, which is one of the reasons it is important to sleep in a dark room.
- TSH (Thyrotropin Stimulating Hormone), which is critical to our metabolism, is released during the onset of sleep and is controlled by our circadian clock.
- Parathyroid hormone release (also important to metabolism) increases during sleep.
- Prolactin is released during the first third of the night, during Delta wave sleep.
- Corticotrophin Releasing Factor is also controlled and released by the pituitary during sleep.
- TRF (Thyrotropin Releasing Factor), another substance related to metabolism, is secreted during sleep.

- VIP (Vasoactive Intestinal Peptide) is released during sleep.

- Leptin, a hormone which regulates the amount of fat storage in your body, is released almost exclusively during sleep. Sleep deprivation results in low levels of leptin, which stimulates your body to increase fat storage and makes you feel hungry, even if your body does not need food.

- Cortisol is released during the end stages of sleep, and is believed to be part of the waking process. Abnormally high levels of cortisol have been linked to memory impairment, stress, insulin resistance and obesity. So if sleep cycles are abnormal, or you are sleep deprived, the resulting high levels of cortisol can wreak havoc with your body.

- ACTH, also involved in metabolic process, is regulated by circadian rhythm.

- DHEA is secreted by the adrenal gland and is a precursor or source ingredient to virtually every hormone your body needs. DHEA production INCREASES UP TO 90% during Theta and Delta wave activity.

- Serotonin may be released during alpha wave activity during the onset of sleep, and may facilitate sleep when released. Tryptophan, the precursor to Serotonin, may facilitate Serotonin release and sleep.

- Glucose metabolism can be profoundly affected by sleep deprivation. Lack of sleep severely decreases your ability to regulate glucose, resulting in abnormally high glucose levels AND a decrease in insulin production. **High glucose levels will, without question, cause weight gain.**

No matter what science does or does not understand about sleep, it is clear from these facts that an adequate amount of high quality nightly sleep is **CRITICAL** to our health and the weight management process.

CIRCIDIAN RHYTHM

Circadian rhythm is the daily 24 hour light/dark cycle which regulates virtually everything about our body and the bodies of all mammals, profoundly affecting our health, our wellbeing, AND OUR WEIGHT. Circadian comes from the Latin Root circa, meaning "about" and Diem meaning "day". Insuring that your circadian rhythm is operating the way nature intended is critical to weight management.

Medical scientists may not know everything (or even close to everything) about exactly HOW sleep and circadian rhythm affects our weight or exactly WHY they affect our weight so profoundly. But they know enough, and yet they say nothing – or next to nothing. Why hasn't anybody galloped through the streets nailing up proclamations and shouting a warning?

Obviously none of them are willing to go out on a limb and even attempt to provide this information in a way that would be meaningful or seem significant to those of us who have serious weight management problems. Why? Because, since they don't know everything, and so much is still unknown – especially the why – they are afraid that decades from now some researcher will discover something that makes some minor detail of their premature pronouncement incorrect and that they might consequently look less than brilliant to their colleagues. Never mind that the rest of us might have organized a religion around their wisdom and paid homage to them in the interim! Where is Paul Revere when you need him?

I, on the other hand, am not afraid of the limb. In fact, I love the limb, I embrace the limb. So hear this:

EVERYTHING you can do to INSURE your CIRCIDIAN CYCLE is NORMAL is CRUCIAL to BOTH your WEIGHT AND your OVERALL HEALTH

The information about circadian rhythm presented in this section is every bit as important as the foregoing information about sleep. In fact, circadian rhythm is so closely interrelated with sleep that the two are as tightly bound as you and your shadow.

The single most important thing I can tell you about circadian rhythm is this:

In October 2010 Ohio State University researchers published a study wherein mice that were forced to artificially experienced an ABNORMAL day/night (circadian) cycle because they were exposed ONLY to DIM LIGHT (rather than complete darkness) at night, GAINED FIFTY PERCENT MORE WEIGHT than the other group of mice that experienced a standard day/night (circadian) cycle with normal dark at night. During the two months of the study all other conditions experienced by the two groups of mice were the same. Both groups ate the same amount of food and had similar activity levels.

According to the researchers the group of mice that was exposed to the dim light at night began eating at unnatural times when their digestive systems were not keyed to metabolize food.

It is beyond my comprehension why the published research did NOT go on and discuss the fact that clearly essential hormones and chemicals produced by the body based on circadian cycles and sleep were either NOT released OR were released in abnormal quantities due to the dim light that prevented the little mousey circadian rhythms from functioning properly. But it seems pretty clear to me that was the case.

This fact alone should be enough to motivate you to do whatever you can to cater to your body's circadian cycle needs. But in case you need more motivation, let me tell you a few more important facts.

Disruption of the normal circadian cycle will cause the suppression or complete blockage of the release of melatonin, other essential hormones, and disrupts thousands of genes in the circadian gene network. THIS CAN RESULT IN:

- **WEIGHT GAIN AND OBESITY**
- Release of excess leptin which causes the body to store excess fat, and prompts excessive hunger.
- Hyperlipidemia
- Hyperglycemia (high levels of sugar in the blood which causes rapid weight gain)
- Lower insulin production
- Insulin resistance
- Onset of Metabolic Syndrome
- High Cholesterol
- Type 2 Diabetes
- Post menopausal osteoporosis
- Certain types of cancer including breast cancer, lung cancer, renal cell carcinoma and brain tumors
- Coronary Heart Disease
- Epilepsy
- Multiple sclerosis

This information should be strongly motivating to take steps to insure your circadian rhythm is regular and normal.

Research studies show that at least ten percent, and maybe more, of our genes are exclusively cued to ***operate*** *ONLY* by ***OR*** are cued to ***operate correctly ONLY*** by the daily shifts between light and dark. The genes ***KNOWN*** to be affected by our Circadian rhythm control some of our most basic bodily functions. Some of the most fascinating facts currently known by medical science are:

- Some medications actually work more effectively if taken at certain times of day. For instance, thyroid medications are most effective if taken shortly before bedtime, unless your doctor has advised you otherwise.

- Sleep cycles, heartbeat, blood pressure, liver and kidney function, body temperature, hormonal changes and even cognitive abilities all clearly show control by circadian rhythm.

- In August 2010 a study was published showing that countries generating the highest levels of light at night also had the highest rates of breast cancer.

    - This is particularly interesting because it has only been in the past 100 years or so that artificial electric light has affected a large percentage of the population.

    - In fact, outside of major metropolitan centers such as New York, London, Paris, etc., artificial light at night probably didn't become an issue in most parts of the world until 50 years or so ago.

- The World Health Organization has classified shift work as a possible carcinogen, due to the prolific problems suffered by those forced to work when their bodies should be sleeping during the dark of the night.

- Our bodies can be so sensitive to changes in our schedules that in Spring, the change to day light savings time causes heart attacks to spike by as much as 24%.
- Even natural births and deaths show a circadian influence and peak in the early morning hours.

MEASURES YOU SHOULD TAKE TO INSURE NATURAL CIRCIDIAN RHYTHM CYCLES AND ENHANCE YOUR NATURAL SLEEP CYCLE

- Make sure your bedroom or sleeping environment is **DARK**. No light should be coming in from windows or other sources. If this is impossible for whatever reason, wear a sleep mask, which can be obtained from many merchants. I believe the best ones are the very light silk ones similar to those given out by the airlines on long international flights, as you can hardly feel them.

- Your sleeping environment should also be cool and quiet.

- Do not keep a TV or a computer or any other device with a lighted screen in your bedroom. Studies show that reading a book with a small book light (NOT a lamp) is much less disruptive of our circadian rhythms than the light from such screens.

- Establish a relaxing nightly ritual you find soothing, such as a bath or reading quietly before going to sleep. An established routine will cue your body to relax and allow drowsiness to occur.

- Go to bed at a reasonable hour that is consistent on a fairly regular basis (10:00 or 11:00 PM). Studies have shown that the groups who suffer the most devastating consequences of disrupted circadian rhythm are individuals for whom it is impossible to establish a regular nightly schedule of sleep, such as shift workers, medical personnel, students and frequent travelers who suffer from jet lag.

- If you have to go to the bathroom during the night, try to go in the dark. If that is impossible, keep a small flashlight or LED keychain light by the bed and use that to light your way. The dim light is less disruptive to our circadian rhythm than turning on a light that floods the entire room or area

- **EAT BREAKFAST WITHIN 60 MINUTES** of getting up in the morning. ONE OF THE NUMEROUS REASONS breakfast is important is that this meal signals our body (and our circadian rhythm) that our day is starting.

- Sunlight in the morning is a positive factor. Also, if you work indoors, try to increase your exposure to sunlight by working near a window if possible.

- Try to complete exercise or workout routines at least 3 hours before bedtime, so your body has time to relax.

- It is important to finish dinner at least two hours before bedtime so your body can complete the digestive process before you go to sleep.

- Insure that your bed has a good quality, comfortable sleeping surface that is not too hard (many people purchase mattresses that are harder than they should be under the mis-guided notion that this is good for them). It is important that the mattress surface has sufficient room for you and any sleeping companions (including pets) to move around during the night.

Doing what you can to follow these recommendations on a regular basis should result in re-setting and positive maintenance of good circadian rhythm.

A BUTTERFLY FLAPS ITS WINGS IN DENVER CAUSING A TSUNAMI IN JAPAN *(Thyroid, Adrenal and Metabolic Disorders)*

The thyroid gland is a small butterfly-shaped organ located in your neck, just below where an Adam's Apple would be. This tiny, innocuous organ is actually the Mother Control Center of your body. It controls every organ, every system, every single **cell** in your entire body. The slightest malfunction of this tiny butterfly-shaped Mothership can wreak so much havoc throughout your system, it can have the effect of a tsunami on your body.

When functioning properly, a healthy thyroid gland is brimming with iodine-rich protein called thymoglobulin, as well as thyroid hormones thyroxine (T4), triiodothyronine (T3), diothyronine (T2), monoiodothyroanine (T1), and calcitonin. The primary function of these hormones is to regulate your metabolism by controlling the rate at which every cell in your body converts oxygen and calories to energy. **The metablolic rate of *EVERY SINGLE CELL* in the human body is regulated by these hormones, the most important of which is the T3 hormone.**

The most common disorders that fall into this category are fairly limited in number, but if you have any one (or more) of them, it is ***catastrophically detrimental*** to your health and your weight.

THYROID DISORDERS INCLUDE
(but are not limited to)

- Hypothyroidism
- Metabolic Syndrome (a sub-clinical variety of hypothyroidism)
- Hashimoto's Disease
- Hyperthyroidism
- Grave's Disease

ADRENAL DISORDERS INCLUDE
(but are not limited to)

- Adrenal Fatigue
- Adrenal Deficiency

METABOLISM DISORDERS INCLUDE
(but are not limited to)

- Sluggish Metabolism
- Gaucher's Disease

Every one of the listed disorders are some of the most commonly ***undiagnosed or mis-diagnosed*** conditions on earth. Yet these disorders cause ***devastating*** consequences for those who have them. I will hazard a guess that more than 50% of the people who read this book have one of these conditions and don't know it. Hypothyroidism is the most common of all these disorders.

Sadly, obtaining a proper diagnosis if you have any of these disorders can be a challenge. Doctors aren't even taught much about metabolism disorders, including thyroid disorders, anymore. Prior to the 1970's common practice was to diagnose metabolism disorders, especially thyroid disorders, by symptoms and then to determine appropriate dosage of medication by the elimination of symptoms; increasing the dosage of medication until all symptoms were gone and the patient felt good. Doctors used lab tests only to confirm what they already knew, **not** as the only legitimate diagnostic tool.

It is not only unfortunate, but, given the track record of the FDA, more than a little suspicious, that since Synthroid and other Synthetic T4 medications came on the market in the late 1950's, a misguided "one size fits all" approach has prevailed in the diagnosis of thyroid disorders, especially Hypothyroidism.

Today, doctors act as if the results of a few simple blood tests are Holy Scripture handed down by God Almighty, regardless of any symptoms you may be suffering. The fact that the reference ranges for these blood tests vary from lab to lab, and the fact that the established reference ranges are highly questionable to begin with is completely ignored.

Most doctors today don't even recognize the majority of the symptoms of metabolic disorders as being associated with a metabolic problem. If you have any metabolic disorder, there are many doctors who will run a few tests, tell you there is nothing wrong with you, and that the symptoms you are suffering are all in your head. Further, many people have more than one metabolic disorder, because these types of disorders have cascade effects and one may trigger another. Such as cases where ongoing, undiagnosed, untreated Hypothyroidism causes Adrenal Fatigue.

To further complicate matters, in many instances a metabolic disorder may actually be the initial root cause of obesity issues and a metabolic disorder combined with obesity may cause a sleep disorder. But a sleep disorder, especially a long term one, can wreak such havoc with your endocrinal system that sleep disorders may trigger a metabolic disorder.

Further, if you have BOTH a metabolic disorder and a sleep disorder, regardless of the order in which they occurred, solving one will ***NOT*** necessarily resolve the other. You ***MUST*** have both diagnosed and have treatment for both. Now perhaps you understand my chicken or egg dilemma!

For years I have had doctors diagnose my thyroid and metabolic disorders incorrectly, treating symptoms as standalone health problems with ***ZERO*** recognition of the fact that these issues were all symptoms of a metabolic disorder. ***OR***, even worse for my mental health, often when the doctor couldn't solve the problem due to their own incompetence or ignorance, they became defensive and acted as if I were making the whole thing up. Of course I am saying this with the benefit of 20/20 hindsight. Knowing what I know now, it is clear to me that my thyroid disorder began before age 7; who knows, I may have been born with it.

If this has happened to you, rest assured you aren't crazy! You have medical problems. The important thing is to find a doctor who understands these types of disorders and will work with you to discover solutions. Consider this fair warning, you may have to drive further than your nearest medical complex to find this enlightened, compassionate, knowledgeable, unconventional physician.

THYROID DISORDERS

Experts estimate that 60 Million people in the United States alone have ***undiagnosed*** Thyroid Disorders. I believe the number is **far** higher, ***at least 50% to 100% higher than this estimate***.

Even among those who ***DO*** have a diagnosed Thyroid Disorder, most are ***not*** receiving effective treatment and continue to have numerous symptoms the patient themselves may not even recognize as being associated with their Thyroid Disorder.

Too many people go through life believing that doctors are Gods, or at least talk to him daily. Not only are doctors ***NOT*** gods, many of them are arrogant, unsympathetic, lazy, greedy, authoritarians who view medicine as a business and patients as profit centers (an attitude encouraged and proliferated by today's medical insurance companies). If your condition requires too much time and attention (making you less profitable) many doctors will slap a label on your problem, issue a prescription or a treatment with no concern as to the appropriateness, and move on to the patients who require less effort – this practice is highly motivated and sustained by today's insurance reimbursement procedures. There is actually a strong movement in the medical community to refuse to treat obese patients; obese patients have been classified "high risk" by the medical community in order to make this practice appear more politically correct.

However, even doctors who are good people that care and go above and beyond to help you, may not be well educated in the area of Thyroid Disorders and Metabolic problems. This is not surprising, since most medical schools today do not teach students much of anything about these issues except interpreting lab results.

It is up to you to educate yourself, and take an active role in your own healthcare. You must prepare for medical visits. Be ready to offer FIRM "suggestions" to the physician as to what may be wrong, why you believe your assessment is correct, and what medications or treatments you believe might be beneficial. It is also important to actually listen to what the doctor says, ***MAKE NOTES***, research what they have contributed to the conversation, and form your own opinion regarding what path you believe your diagnosis and treatment should take. If the doctor doesn't agree with you, you can ***EITHER*** find another doctor, ***OR*** try things the way the doctor wants to do them. If your symptoms persist, ***THEN*** find another doctor.

Many people give up due to the high cost of going from doctor to doctor in order to get a proper diagnosis. Once you have a proper diagnosis and the correct treatment, insurance will cover the majority of the cost. Consequently it is important to research doctors you believe may be helpful before you make an appointment.

HYPOTHYROIDISM

Hypothyroidism (**Underactive** Thyroid) is a condition where your thyroid gland doesn't produce sufficient thyroid hormones. Hypothyroidism results in a devastating imbalance in the chemical reactions that drive every cell in your entire body. Over time, hypothyroidism causes numerous serious or even fatal health problems. Hypothyroidism is one of the most under-diagnosed, misdiagnosed, untreated, undertreated, and unidentified or undetected medical conditions in the world. Of the 60 to 120+ million people in the U.S. alone with undiagnosed Thyroid Disorders, I'm going to go out on a limb (loving the limb!) and estimate that over 90% of those people have Hypothyroidism or Metabolic Syndrome, or both. Further, most of those with undiagnosed Hypothyroidism are women, as Hypothyroidism occurs 5 times more frequently in women than men.

An alarmingly high percentage of people with Hypothyroidism are misdiagnosed as having completely different conditions. Usually when this happens, a **symptom** of Hypothyroidism is diagnosed as the primary condition. Some of the most commonly misdiagnosed patients are labeled with depression and given mood altering medications such as Prozac or Xanax; coronary diseases are mis-diagnosed as the primary condition and treated independently; fatigue and low energy issues are labeled as "designer" conditions such as Chronic Fatigue or Epstein-Barr Syndrome and treated accordingly; aches and pains are mis-diagnosed as arthritis (or juvenile arthritis in younger people) and treated with NSAIDS; and obese patients who can't lose weight are labeled as overeaters and treated appallingly.

This mind-boggling list could go on and on. Sadly, since these patients are being incorrectly treated and their symptoms continue to persist, many of them are labeled cranks, hypochondriacs or told it is all in their head and they are dismissed as hysterical women. The only thing any of these poor, mistreated souls need is thyroid medication to clear up their problems.

The vast majority of people reading this book probably have Hypothyroidism, whether or not you have been diagnosed. Even if you ***have*** been diagnosed with Hypothyroidism, there is a good chance you are ***NOT*** on the correct medication. Even if you ***ARE*** on the correct medication, your dosage may be incorrect. The results of a study published in November 2010 showed over 37% of **diagnosed** Hypothyroid patients receiving treatment ***were receiving an incorrect dose of medication***, most were receiving **insufficient** dosages.

Doctors commonly run only two or three blood tests, and use the results of those tests as their ***only*** diagnostic tool. Unfortunately, blood work won't tell them much. Even ***IF*** the blood work was the holy grail of diagnostic tools, the reference ranges utilized by labs to categorize "normal" results are at the very least questionable. Many experts believe the reference ranges for thyroid tests are completely wrong.

For instance, Thyroid Stimulating Hormone, or "TSH", is the most common test misguidedly used to diagnose a thyroid condition. Your pituitary produces TSH to tell your thyroid to produce thyroid hormones. If your TSH is high it means your thyroid is not producing enough thyroid hormones and your pituitary is sending frantic "send more hormones" messages. You have Hypothyroidism. However, most labs today set the "normal" reference range for TSH from as low as 0.3 to as high as 6.0! This is a **huge** reference range.

For some reason most doctors seem to be biased AGAINST issuing a Hypothyroidism diagnosis, even if you have severe hypothyroid symptoms. Your thyroid blood test results could come back with every single test showing you are on the extreme end of the "normal" reference range, and your doctor will **still** tell you that you are fine. Worse, even ***IF*** the blood work shows that you are clearly Hypothyroid, the results certainly don't indicate what medication will work best to treat your problem.

Whether you know very little or a great deal about Hypothyroidism, you may find the list of symptoms/side effects of Hypothyroidism below shocking. I bet there are things on this list you never even imagined were symptoms of a thyroid problem. With something as pervasive as Hypothyroidism, which frequently goes undiagnosed for years, it is extremely difficult to separate the symptoms from the side effects, so there is only one single list below encompassing both.

You may have Hypothyroidism even if you have NONE of the problems on the list because symptoms of Hypothyroidism arise slowly and gradually worsen over time. However, if you have five or more of the following list of symptoms, you almost certainly have Hypothyroidism.

SYMPTOMS/SIDE EFFECTS OF HYPOTHYROIDISM INCLUDE
(but are not limited to)

- **UNEXPLAINED CHRONIC WEIGHT GAIN**
- **INABILITY TO LOSE WEIGHT**

- **OBESITY OR MORBID OBESITY**
- Chronic Fatigue
- Sluggishness
- Low Energy
- Low Stamina
- Nodding off easily
- Requiring afternoon naps
- Sleep Apnea
- Insomnia
- Sensitivity to room temperature (always feeling cold or hot)
- Cold hands or feet even when warm
- Pale, dry skin
- Skin so dry it feels like "snake" skin
- Peeling skin
- Paresthesia (tingling or crawling of the skin)
- Brittle hair and fingernails
- Broken/peeling fingernails
- Dry hair
- Coarse hair
- Hair loss or thin hair
- No eyebrows or thin eyebrows

- Abnormal body temperature (chronic temperature ABOVE or BELOW 98.6 – temperature may even fluctuate between the two extremes)
- Chronic headaches and/or migraines
- Inability to concentrate
- Forgetfulness
- "Foggy" thinking
- Difficulty recalling names
- Delayed or slow cognitive processing of information
- Decreased speed of sensory and cognitive processing
- Impaired or altered cognitive function
- Irritability/Extreme Irritability
- Intolerance of others
- Exhaustion – physical, mental, or emotional
- Panic Attacks
- Post-Traumatic Stress Disorder (PTSD) like symptoms
- Chronic low grade depression
- Depression (Hypothyroidism is frequently misdiagnosed as depression)
- Suicidal thoughts
- Dementia
- Inability to have a relationship with anyone

- Impaired or non-existent sex drive
- Muscle aches
- Muscular tenderness and stiffness
- Muscle weakness
- Muscle cramps and charley horses
- Pain or swelling in joints
- Joint stiffness
- Osteoporosis
- Unable to stand on feet for long periods
- Sore feet, plantar fasciitis, painful soles of feet
- Carpal tunnel symptoms
- Aching bones/muscles
- Swelling/edema/puffiness
- Puffy face
- Swollen legs that prevent walking
- Fluid retention
- Long recovery period requited after an activity
- Exercise causes severe debilitation and exhaustion
- Arms feel like dead weights after activity
- Slowing to a snail's pace when walking up hill
- Complete lack of motivation

- Inability to work full time
- Sensitivity to being in the sun
- Sunburns regardless of using sun block after even a short time in the sun
- Exhaustion, nausea or dizziness after being in sun
- Allergies (which may result from low cortisol)
- Tightness in throat, sore throat
- Hoarse voice
- Swollen lymph glands
- Decreased motility of the esophagus
- Difficulty swallowing
- Heartburn
- Acid Reflux
- Dysphasia, which is the inability to swallow fluid, food, pills, or your own saliva
- Dizziness and vertigo from fluid on the inner ear
- Ringing in the ears
- Internal itching of the ears
- High total cholesterol – Hypothyroidism is one of the leading causes of high cholesterol; yet millions of people with TSH at the highest end of the "normal" reference range are taking expensive statins. If all the undiagnosed or undertreated cases of hypothyroidism

were diagnosed and treated properly would statin drugs even be necessary? Surely they would be less prevalent.)

- Decreased LDL (good cholesterol)
- Hardening of the arteries
- Arterial plaque build up
- Palpitations of the Heart
- Fibrillations
- Cardiovascular Disease – individuals suffering from hypothyroidism are 3.4 times MORE likely to develop Cardiovascular Disease.
- Congestive Heart Failure
- Chronic Elevated or severely elevated C-Reactive Protein (CRP) with no explanation
- Blood pressure problems
- Hypertension
- Varicose Veins
- Extreme hunger, especially at night, or in the middle of the night
- Inability to eat in the mornings
- No Appetite
- Lactose Intolerance
- Indigestion
- Nausea

- Vomiting
- Anxious Bladder
- Painful Bladder
- Abdominal discomfort
- Flatulence and bloating
- Hard Stools
- Decreased motility of the bowels
- Constipation
- Colitis
- Irritable Bowel Syndrome
- Intestinal Obstruction
- Abnormal enlargement of the colon
- Severe PMS
- Moody Periods
- Excruciating pain/cramps during period
- Heavy menstrual periods
- Constant or abnormally frequent menstrual spotting or bleeding
- Failure to ovulate
- Inability to get pregnant
- Miscarriages
- Acne on face and in hair

- Breakout on chest and arms
- Bumps on legs
- Hives

Hypothyroidism signs and symptoms build up and become more severe over time if left untreated. Myxedema (or severely advanced hypothyroidism) is a rare, but life-threatening condition. Symptoms include low blood pressure, shallow breathing, decreased body temperature, unresponsiveness and even coma. In extreme cases, myxedema can be fatal.

The best determination of whether or not you have Hypothyroidism will be the number of symptoms you have, and how many of those symptoms are eliminated over time after you begin taking thyroid medication. While lab work is not the holy grail of diagnostic tools for Hypothyroidism, and lab results should be viewed with some level of skepticism, it is still a good idea to have a complete panel of thyroid blood work done. Most doctors won't prescribe medication without the labs anyway. You should also be aware that results of these tests can vary based on time of day, stress, sleep, day of week, and other factors. So you may be told you're fine based on lab work today, but show severe thyroid problems tomorrow. Insist that your doctor run ALL of the following tests:

- TSH (Thyroid Stimulating Hormone) test
- Total T4
- Free T4
- Total T3

- Free T3
- Reverse T3
- Autoimmune antibodies (TPOAb – see Hashimoto's)

Some other tests that can be run, but which are not common and might not be covered by insurance are:

- Biopsy or Enzymatic Studies of the Thyroid Gland
- Ultrasound or Scintigraphy
- HPA (Hypothalamic Pituitary Axis) test

There is a great deal of confusing information available on numerous medical sites regarding results of thyroid lab tests and how to interpret them. As I have noted, the "normal" reference ranges used by most labs are fairly useless. Following are the optimal reference ranges recommended by some of the maverick experts:

- TSH – Use reference range 0.2 to 2.0 mIU/L.
    - If your TSH is over 2.0, you should be on thyroid medication.
    - If your TSH is over 3.0 you have a significant case of Hypothyroidism.
    - If your TSH is over 4.0 you have significant Hypothyroidism and you are at high risk for cardiovascular problems.

- ***If you are overweight, you want your TSH to be as close to 0.2 mIU/L as possible OR even lower.***

- TSH below 0.2 is technically considered to be **Hyper**thyroid (which, medically speaking, means your thyroid is over active). Doctors used to believe that TSH below 0.2 caused loss of bone density; however ***THIS HAS BEEN DISPROVEN BY MEDICAL STUDY AFTER MEDICAL STUDY***. The best study I have seen published in 2011 followed scores of patients for two decades, medicating those patients to TSH as low as 0.0001 mIU/L with no loss of bone density and no harmful side effects. The results of this and several other studies published over the last 15 years prove conclusively that doctors ***SHOULD*** be medicating patients with gradually increasing doses of thyroid medication until all their symptoms are eliminated (including obesity) and their patients feel well, regardless of a TSH level that goes below the low end of the "normal" reference range.

Many doctors are unaware of these facts, and refuse to prescribe medication even for patients who have TSH at the very highest end of the "normal" reference range, regardless of the severity of the Hypothyroid symptoms the patient is suffering.

- Total T4 isn't usually a very important test, but the reference range you should utilize is 8.0 to 12.0 mcg/dL (micrograms per deciliter). Most labs use 4.5 to 12.0 as the "normal" reference range, but you should be in the upper end of the range (close to 12.0), especially if you have a weight problem.

- Free T4 – the reference range you should use is 1.2 to 1.53 ng/dL (nanograms per deciliter). Labs commonly use 0.70 to 1.53 ng/dL. Anything under 1.2 ng/dL is too low.

- Total T3 – this test is of more value. The reference range you should use is 120-140 to 180-200 ng/mL (nanograms per milliliter). Labs commonly use 60-100 to 180-200 ng/mL. Anything under 120-140 is too low.

- Free T3 is the most critical test. The optimal reference range is 420 to 480 pg/mL (pictograms per milliliter). Most labs use 260 to 480 pg/mL. (OR if the labs reference range is 2.0 to 4.5, you want your bloodwork to be in the 4.0 to 4.5 range.)

- Reverse T3 – If your reverse T3 is ABOVE the optimal reference range of 90 to 150 pg/mL, your body is blocking your T3 and you need medication. Labs commonly use 90 to 350 pg/mL as the "normal" reference range. Anything over 150 pg/mL is too high.

METABOLIC SYNDROME

Metabolic Syndrome is a disorder of energy utilization and storage that is related to Hypothyroidism. Metabolic Syndrome was only identified by the medical community less than 20 years ago, and is still rarely diagnosed. It is diagnosed based on these five risk factors, Large Waist Size, High Triglycerides, Low HDL (good cholesterol), High Blood

Pressure and High fasting blood sugar. If you have three of these five conditions, you have Metabolic Syndrome. People with Metabolic Syndrome are twice as likely to have a heart attack or a stroke, and nearly five times more likely to have Diabetes Type 2.

I myself have been diagnosed with Metabolic Syndrome. If you have Metabolic Syndrome, you may suffer SOME or MANY of the symptoms of hypothyroidism listed previously. It is highly likely that patients with Metabolic Syndrome ALSO have Hypothyroidism. ADDITIONAL symptoms of Metabolic Syndrome include:

SYMPTOMS OF METABOLIC SYNDROME INCLUDE

(but are not limited to)

- **OBESITY OR MORBID OBESITY**
- **Carrying a majority of your weight around the core or center of your body**
- **INABILITY TO LOSE WEIGHT regardless of diet or exercise**
- Diabetes Type 2
- Insulin Resistant
- High Triglycerides
- High Blood Pressure
- Common thyroid dysfunction blood tests may appear normal

The treatment for Metabolic Syndrome is the same as for Hypothyroidism, and patients will take hypothyroid medications.

HASHIMOTO'S DISEASE

If you have Hashimoto's Disease, getting a correct diagnosis can be unbelievably difficult unless you at least suspect Hashimoto's is your problem and insist the doctor test for it up front. Regular thyroid blood work (questionable as it is) will almost never be indicative of Hashimoto's and in fact will hinder rather than help to get to the correct diagnosis in most cases.

Hashimoto's Thyroiditis is actually an autoimmune condition. If you have Hashimoto's it means your thyroid gland is being attacked by antibodies in your blood, which will eventually destroy the thyroid gland and its ability to function. If this occurs, you will have permanent Hypothyroidism.

The reason this condition is so difficult to diagnose is because the attacks on your thyroid may cause bursts of over activity on the part of your thyroid gland. This causes thyroid blood work to indicate you are Hypothyroid sometimes, and Hyperthyroid other times in a whiplash effect. So if blood tests are run day after day, you may test Hypothyroid one day, and Hyperthyroid the next, while on other days your blood work may appear normal, as if you have no thyroid issue at all.

If you have Hashimoto's the only way to diagnose it is by the two antibody lab tests called:

- Anti-TPO; and
- TgAb

Patients who suffer from Hashimoto's Disease may not have any symptoms in the beginning, but will usually eventually display some of the symptoms of Hypothyroidism. They may also display any of the following additional symptoms and side effects:

SYMPTOMS/SIDE EFFECT OF HASHIMOTO'S DISEASE INCLUDE *(but are not limited to)*

- ANY/ALL symptoms/side effects of Hypothyroidism
- Sore throat
- Tightness in throat
- Discomfort wearing a turtleneck or any shirt that is snug at the neck
- Difficulty swallowing
- Goiter
- Possible symptoms of Hyperthyroid

Treatment of Hashimoto's Disease is currently for patients to take Hypothyroid medications. There have been recent studies that suggest that even with Hypothyroid medication, Hashimoto's patients continue to suffer lingering symptoms.

HYPOTHYROID MEDICATIONS

Once you are finally diagnosed with Hypothyroidism of any kind, the treatment is prescription thyroid medication. However, not all thyroid medications are created equal.

For reasons known only to the FDA, Knoll Pharmaceutical Company (the pharmaceutical that first created it), and whoever got rich because of it, Synthoid is the most commonly prescribed thyroid medication for Hypothyroidism in the United States, and most of the world. Synthroid is **nothing** but **Synthetic** T4. Synthroid was the first synthetic thyroid medication (then known as Levothyroixine Sodium) to come on the market back in 1955. The generic equivalent is Levothyroixine, and there are several other brand names of this medication including Lovoxyl, Unithroid, Oroxine and Eltroxin. Nearly 100% of newly diagnosed cases of Hypothyroidism are treated with prescription Synthroid or other brands of Synthetic T4. ***Don't let your doctor do this to you!!***

Why synthetic? A very intelligent question. Where hormones are concerned, isn't natural better? Ah, my dear Watson, a very astute observation! My response would be ***YES***, natural is better. Read on.

Many individuals with Hypothyroidism actually have the problem that their bodies don't properly or effectively convert T4 to T3. In these cases the patient, who has initially been prescribed a Synthetic T4 medication, continues to suffer symptoms while taking the Synthetic T4 until the physician determines this additional information (**IF** they ever do discover it). Once discovered, the patient is then frequently switched to a Synthetic T3, such as Cytomel, Tertroxin or

Cynomel. But, taking ONLY Synthetic T3 can create the same types of imbalances as taking only Synthetic T4.

Sometimes doctors try combining a prescription for Synthetic T4 together with a prescription for Synthetic T3. However getting the balance correct can prove to be nightmarish for the patient and almost never achieves the desired result. There is one Synthetic T4/T3 combination available by the name of Thyrolar, although it has to be refrigerated and therefore can cause difficulties for those who travel, and it is ***still*** synthetic.

My advice? SKIP ALL the synthetic drugs, the problems they create, and waiting additional months or years or forever to actually start feeling better. Go directly to the best type of medication on the market, a tried and true natural pharmaceutical, Natural Desiccated Thyroid medication.

Due to ignorant, incompetent doctors, it took me 30 years to discover the joys of this type of medication which ultimately not only worked the best for me – it actually changed my life. For 30 years I actually believed all the hooey doctors parrot like trained myna birds: *"thyroid medication won't cause weight loss; depression isn't a symptom of thyroid problems; your joints hurt because you have orthopedic problems; you have fibromyalgia; migraines aren't caused by thyroid problems;"* and on and on. Once I started taking Armour Thyroid ***ALL*** my symptoms miraculously started clearing up and I lost weight for the first time in more than a decade, ***because my thyroid was FINALLY WORKING NORMALLY!***

There is a growing movement among thyroid patients for Natural Desiccated Thyroid medication. This type of medication was originally developed in the late 1800's compounded from desiccated porcine thyroid. These were the original medications utilized to control Hypothyroidism, have enjoyed *CONTINUOUS FDA APPROVAL* for nearly a century, and have proven to be extremely effective for more than 100 years. Natural Desiccated Thyroid medication has the advantage of containing *ALL* of the thyroid hormones, T4, T3, T2, T1, and calcitonin, in a balance that is virtually identical to the thyroid hormones produced naturally by a healthy human thyroid. These types of medication are still compounded from porcine thyroid and are sold under many brand names, including:

- Armour Thyroid (the most well known U.S. brand)
- Naturethroid (another U.S. brand)
- Westhroid (another U.S. brand)
- Acella (a generic) and other generic brands
- Thyroid-S or Thiroyd (a relatively new entrant from Thailand)
- Erfa's Thyroid (from Canada)
- Cenetic (from Italy)
- Thyreolgland (from Germany)
- Thyreoidum (from Denmark)
- And compounded Desiccated Thyroid Powder from Australia

Proponents of Natural Desiccated Thyroid medications point out that it is far superior to synthetic pharmaceuticals due to the fact that it is completely natural. It contains ALL of the same thyroid hormones that should be produced by your body in proportions nearly identical to a healthy, well functioning human thyroid. And because it is natural your body accepts ALL of the medication's natural components (unless you have an allergy to porcine). So of course it is better!

Astonishingly, many doctors today have never even heard of Natural Desiccated Thyroid medications. Unbelievably, some pharmaceutical reference books and databases don't even list these medications. Many doctors will tell you that these medications are outdated, have gone off the market, are unstable, or even claim that they are dangerous; asserting that they have been replaced with "better", "modern" (synthetic and more expensive) pharmaceuticals. All this means is that some pharmaceutical company is growing rich because they can charge far more for an engineered synthetic medication they have "invented" than you pay for something natural. And the insurance company or the doctor or both are lining their pockets with "bonuses" (bribes) paid to them by the pharmaceutical company for prescribing these more expensive synthetic medications that leave the majority of patients undertreated and miserable. Don't believe me? Read the information in the chapter about Medical Insurance and Doctors.

Most Natural Desiccated Thyroid medications are ***LESS THAN HALF THE COST*** of any synthetic thyroid medication. Insist your doctors prescribe a Natural Desiccated Thyroid medication for you FROM THE BEGINNING, OR find another doctor.

See the strategies at the end of this chapter for assistance in finding a doctor in your area who is familiar with the benefits of and prescribes Natural Desiccated Thyroid medication for their patients. Actually, unless you adore your current doctor, you might be best served by finding one of these doctors to diagnose your thyroid condition.

What is the proper dosage of thyroid medication? When ALL your symptoms are eliminated and you feel good, you are on the correct dose. When your doctor first prescribes thyroid medication for you, allow a month or so to go by and see how you feel – the dosage of your medication should be gradually increased every few weeks until ALL of your symptoms have been eliminated. Don't allow your doctor to stop increasing your dosage, until you find that you are not only feeling well, but that ALL your symptoms have been eliminated.

If there were even a shred of doubt in my mind about the efficacy of Armour Thyroid and how it changed my life, it was proven to me in no uncertain terms that Synthetic T4 medications are useless or worse than useless when a new doctor refused to prescribe anything other than Synthroid. Within two weeks of this change, I started having serious hypothyroid symptoms. The doctor claimed that as long as my TSH was within the normal range (anywhere within the normal range) I was fine, and any symptoms I reported experiencing were imaginary.

Of course, I wasn't fine at all. I was miserable. And, to make matters worse, I started gaining back the weight I had lost. When I told the doctor that I was eating approximately 1,100 calories a day, high protein, low carbohydrate, food intake, the doctor told me that was obviously why I was gaining weight, I wasn't eating enough!! In addition to gaining weight, I was once again suffering from insomnia, menstrual problems (despite the fact that I was post-menopausal when I entered prison), chronic headaches, aching muscles and joints, chronic fatigue, dry skin, brittle nails, my cholesterol started going up dramatically, and myriad other problems, all of which had disappeared while I was taking Armour Thyroid. Some of these problems, like the insomnia, I hadn't even ever REALIZED were hypothyroid related.

This experience got me thinking about the dramatic difference in the way my body reacted to Armour Thyroid medication versus Synthetic T4 medication. I have no medical proof (of course), but I started wondering if Synthetic T4 medications actually do ***anything*** besides causing bloodwork to ***appear*** to meet the "normal" criteria?

*HYPER*THYROIDISM AND GRAVE'S DISEASE

It is unlikely that anyone with *Hyper*thyroidism is even reading this book. One of the classic symptoms of *Hyper*thyroidism is the ***INABILITY to GAIN WIEGHT***. I have known people who were *Hyper*thyroid, and it's a little bit obnoxious to listen to them whine about having to drink 5 milkshakes a day and eat all those hamburgers and french fries and hot fudge sundaes when all they really want to do is eat healthy. It's just so hard to be a size zero and not be able to put on any weight!!! They're kidding, right???

But, to be serious, *Hyper*thyroidism is a condition which can result in as many adverse consequences as an underactive thyroid.

If you are *Hyper*thyroid, it means your thyroid gland is producing too much T3. Medications to control *Hyper*thyroidism include methimazole or proplythiouracil.

Graves Disease is noted in some medical journals as being the CAUSE of *Hyper*thyroidism, and in other medical journals is noted as being a more advanced form of *Hyper*thyroidism. Whichever the case, treatment is required which may include Radioactive Iodine, causing destruction of the thyroid gland or in the worst scenario where a very acute case has resulted in thyrotoxicosis (or thyroid storm), surgical removal of the thyroid gland may be necessary. In the event that the thyroid gland must be destroyed or surgically removed, of course this renders the individual Hypothyroid for the rest of their life.

Fortunately *Hyper*thyroidism in all its forms only affects about one percent of the population.

ADRENAL DISORDERS

The two adrenal disorders which primarily relate to Hypothyroidism and weight gain are:

- Adrenal Fatigue
- Adrenal Deficiency

Although you will read about these two topics as if they were two different conditions, for all intents and purposes they are the same condition.

There are two other adrenal disorders which are much more extreme, Addison's Disease and Cushing's Syndrome. In fact, unless you have one of these two much more serious conditions, most doctors don't even discuss adrenal dysfunction as being a medical problem, and rarely do mainstream medical doctors suggest testing for the milder Adrenal Fatigue/Adrenal Deficiency unless prompted or insisted upon by a patient.

ADRENAL FATIGUE/ADRENAL DEFICIENCY

Experts estimate that Adrenal Fatigue or Adrenal Deficiency affect 50% or more of patients with Hypothyroidism, especially those Hypothyroid patients who have gone undiagnosed for an extended period, or those who have been on a Synthetic T4 only regimen for a long period.

Your adrenal glands are walnut-size glands that sit above your kidneys. The adrenals help you cope with stress of all varieties, physical, emotional, or mental. The adrenals are called to action by a communication from the hypothalamus to the pituitary, which in turn triggers the adrenal glands with a hormone called Adrenocorticotropic Hormone (ACTH).

In response to proper stimulation, your adrenals produce hormones, two of which are most important to the issues at hand:

- Aldosterone, which helps maintain your internal fluid balance, blood pressure, sex hormones (testosterone and estrogen), DHEA and others
- Cortisol, which plays a major role in long-term reduction of stress and blood sugar levels. And, very important for thyroid patients, Cortisol helps enable thyroid hormones to pass from your blood into your cells. Adrenal dysfunction can slam the

door on cell reception of thyroid hormones regardless of how much T4 and T3 is flooding your body whether naturally, or as a result of hypothyroid medication.

SYMPTOMS OF ADRENAL FATIGUE/ADRENAL DEFICIENCY
(include, but are not limited to)

- Deficiency OR Overproduction of Cortisol
- Deficiency OR Overproduction of Aldosterone
- Deficiency OR Overproduction of Adrenaline
- Anxiety
- Panic Attacks
- OCD (Obsessive-Compulsive Disorder) tendencies
- Confusion
- Forgetfulness/memory problems
- Inability to cope with stress
- Feeling "tired but wired"
- Impatience or irritability
- Lack of patience
- Chronic mood swings/extreme emotional shifts (bursting into tears suddenly)
- Light headedness

- Shakiness or trembling
- Dizziness/vertigo
- Nearly passing out when you stand up
- Flu like symptoms
- Low immune resistance/frequent infections
- Racing or pounding heart
- Frequent urination
- Trouble sleeping
- Hypoglycemia (low blood sugar)
- Sweating
- Onset of clumsiness (dropping things or bumping into things)
- Craving salt or sugar
- Excessive thirst
- Chronic food allergies

There can be several causes of Adrenal Fatigue/Deficiency including ongoing untreated or improperly treated Hypothyroidism, Fluoride (which actually decreases production of thyroid hormones and was previously utilized to treat *Hyper*thyroidism! And, of course, is by law, in our water), and Chlorine which inhibits the iodine receptors of thyroid hormones.

ADRENAL TESTS

- ACTH Stimulation Test
- Blood Serum Cortisol Test
- 24 Hour Urine Collection Test
- Overnight Metyraphone or Dexamethasone Test

All of these tests have certain disadvantages and may ***NOT*** detect a very real case of adrenal dysfunction.

The treatment for Adrenal Fatigue/Deficiency is generally short term Cortisol supplements. Since Cortisol supplements (in lower strength than prescription strength) are available over-the-counter, if you are convinced that you have an adrenal issue and your doctor isn't diagnosing it, it is always easy to take over-the-counter Cortisol supplements. ***HOWEVER***, it is easy to overdose on cortisol which will only cause a different set of problems. Take a Cortisol supplement for only approximately 8 weeks to help your adrenal glands recover and reset themselves.

METABOLISM DISFUNCTION/SLUGGISH METABOLISM

If you are seriously obese or morbidly obese, you probably have a sluggish metabolism ***in addition*** to Hypothyroidism. The best thing to do is discuss with your doctor the options in prescription medication that will stimulate your metabolism, such as phentermine. Taking over the counter or mail order supplements that promise to stimulate your metabolism is generally a waste of money and could be dangerous due to ingredients in some of these supplements. I am a walking, talking testament to the futility of falling for advertisements that promise results but don't deliver.

GAUCHER'S DISEASE

Gaucher's Disease is caused by a lack of Glucocerebrosidase in your body. While it is important to have your condition diagnosed if you have it, this condition affects a very small percentage of the population, and is not necessarily linked with obesity.

THE CANDYMAN
(Sugar and Sugar Addiction)

There is a substance which is generally either white or brown, it comes primarily in crystallized or powdered form, it is cheap and readily available and ***it is more highly addictive than heroine.*** We needn't worry about maintaining a police presence near schools, playgrounds and places where children congregate to protect them from this addictive, toxic substance, because we ourselves give it to them, with love. I am talking about sugar.

Most medical sources say very politically correct things such as, *"a link has been discovered between sugar and the pleasure centers of the brain which is being studied"* OR *"there is some evidence that sugar may have addictive qualities."* These types of statements are absolute bull puckey!! Let me say it for you again in words that are easy to understand:

SUGAR IS MORE HIGHLY ADDICTIVE THAN HEROINE!!

Sugar is added to most processed food (which is one of the many reasons it is so important to read labels) ***AND*** most restaurant food. Why? ***Because sugar IS so addictive.*** The mega corporations that manufacture and distribute most processed foods want to insure that people will like their product and continue to purchase it. Restaurants want their patrons to come back, over and over again. What is the easiest way to accomplish these goals? Put something in the food that is both legal AND highly addictive.

Sugar (whether listed as sugar, corn syrup, high fructose corn syrup, fructose, dextrose, maltose, lactose, turvinado sugar, date sugar, maple sugar, organic cane syrup or organic cane juice) is present in virtually all processed foods. It is estimated that Americans consume more than 160 POUNDS of sugar and related sweeteners (such as high fructose corn syrup) every year.

A can of non-diet soda contains approximately 17 teaspoons of sugar. Think that carton of fat free yogurt you ate for lunch was healthy? Think again, a 2/3 cup container of flavored yogurt contains on average approximately 7 teaspoons of sugar. Even foods where you would think sugar would be the last thing that should be in there contain sugar. Sugar is added to virtually everything today, catsup, cereal, pancake mix, syrup, bread, salad dressing, peanut butter, pasta, canned and frozen foods and vegetables, luncheon meats, even orange juice. Even some brands of SALT contain sugar!!

Again, READING LABELS IS CRITICAL!

Growing up I loved Campbell's Tomato Soup. It tasted yummy and like tomato soup should taste, tomatoey and a little salty. I hadn't eaten a can of Campbell's Tomato soup in at least a decade due to my acid reflux. Recently I had a cold and got a can of this comfort food for dinner. When I heated the soup and put in a bowl, I was horrified to discover that it tasted like CANDIED TOMATO soup. What happened to my favorite soup? I read the label – 12 GRAMS of sugar were contained in EACH SERVING. According to the label, one can contains 2.5 servings, so there were 30 TOTAL GRAMS of sugar in the soup I was eating; in fact, sugar was the THIRD ingredient in the soup. The soup was inedible and I threw it away – what is sugar doing in tomato soup anyway? Don't tomatoes have enough natural sugar all on their own? But this is an example of how pervasive added sugar has become as an ingredient in processed food.

Due to my weight problems, I made a decision in 1977 to stop eating or drinking processed, refined sugar to the best of my ability. At that time, I started using the only artificial sweetener available on the market, saccharine (or Sweet 'N Low). In spite of the saccharine/cancer scare that happened shortly thereafter, I calculated I would have to drink approximately 40 gallons of soda DAILY to replicate the amount of saccharine being given to the rats to induce cancer – and the 40 gallons of soda would no doubt kill me immediately, saving me the trouble of dying slowly from cancer. I figured I would take my chances with the saccharine. Medical science has since debunked the saccharine/cancer myth and now admits there is no correlation between cancer in humans and saccharine. ***Once again proving me correct!*** (Doesn't everyone love saying "I told you so?")

You might ask, what facts lead you to assert so emphatically that Sugar is addictive? And why hasn't the FDA or any other responsible government agency warned us of these dangers? Both very good questions!

No government agency has seriously warned you about sugar, because of the very lucrative, very rich, very economically powerful, very politically powerful sugar industry. As I have said before, in most cases if you just follow the money, it's pretty easy to figure out.

What makes me assert so emphatically that sugar is as addictive as heroine? Oh, and by the way, refined sugar is **toxic** too.

FACTS ABOUT SUGAR

- Refined sugar is NOT a food. It is a chemical substance. It has NO nutritional value (which is why it is frequently referred to as "empty" calories) and is toxic to your body.
- The brain reacts to sugar almost identically to the way it reacts to heroine. The pleasure center of the brain and neurotransmitters like dopamine and serotonin are stimulated by sugar in the same manner they are stimulated by heroin or cocaine.
- With regular use, tolerance to sugar occurs and it is necessary to increase consumption of sugar to feel the same effects. With regular use, after a period of months, sugar is required for normal functioning.
- In spite of negative consequences (such as weight gain and illness), and even in spite of the desire to give sugar up, people will continue to eat sugar compulsively. Sugar addiction is more difficult to overcome than it is to stop smoking, stop drinking, or kick heroine.

- Physical withdrawal symptoms occur when an addict stops using sugar, such as headaches, irritability, mood swings, sweating, shakiness and light-headedness.
- Frequently eating sugar or sugar addiction may cause aggression and may even lead to a life of crime. According to a recent British study that tracked 17,500 people over decades, 69% of all people convicted of violent crimes ate sweets daily as children. Of those convicted of NON-violent crimes only 42% ate sweets on a daily basis as children.
- Sugar addiction frequently leads to alcoholism or addiction to other drugs such as cocaine or heroin. FURTHER, recovering alcoholics and drug abusers frequently rely on sugar and develop a sugar addiction in order to kick their drug or alcohol habit. You may be shocked to learn that the prison system in the U.S. encourages this by insuring that all inmates have unfettered access to sugar laden foods, desserts and beverages. In most prisons it is nearly impossible for inmates to get access to anything that does NOT contain high quantities of sugar.
- The biochemical composition of refined sugar is identical to alcohol except for one molecule.

Refined sugar is very different, both in chemical composition and the way our body processes it, from naturally occurring sugar found in fruit, some vegetables, and especially honey. Although refined sugar has been around for thousands of years, it was extremely expensive for most of that time. Less than 200 years ago, only the wealthy or the nobility could afford refined sugar with any regularity.

In the 1600s the Venetians began importing large quantities of sugar from the Middle East for the first time and distributed it throughout Europe. But it wasn't until the 1800s that sugar and candies made from refined sugar became affordable and sugar began to be thought of as a household staple. Even then sugar was certainly not consumed in anything approaching the vast quantities most people consume sugar today. This is why many of the degenerative health effects didn't become obvious until the last few decades.

HEALTH PROBLEMS CAUSED BY CONSUMPTION OF REFINED SUGAR

- In order to digest sugar, our body must deplete its reserves of sodium, magnesium, calcium, and potassium to break down and digest the sugar.
- Refined sugar is stored in the liver as glycogen. As the glycogen accumulates in the liver it leads to fatty acids being deposited in the liver, waist, buttocks, belly, thighs, heart, kidneys and other organs.
- In 1957, Dr. William Coda Martin published a study showing that during the digestion of refined sugar a toxic acid is created called pyruvic acid. This acid has a lethal effect on all the cells in our body because it blocks oxygen from getting through to our cells and results in cellular death. You've read how alcohol kills brain cells? Sugar kills cells all over our bodies, and most people consume far more sugar than alcohol. Sugar is by far the more dangerous substance.

- Sugar consumption forces the body to strip calcium from your teeth and bones, resulting in tooth decay, osteoporosis and arthritis.
- Oxygen starvation of brain cells leads to degenerative brain diseases such as Alzheimer's and Dementia.
- Sugar interferes with your body's absorption of protein.
- Obesity
- In your bloodstream sugar converts into 2 to 5 times more fat than starch.
- Diabetes Type 2
- Sugar suppresses the immune system by depleting phagocytes (white blood cells needed for strong immune function and to combat infections and diseases)
- Depletion of the adrenal glands
- Impaired adrenal function
- Candida
- Headaches
- Hypoglycemia
- High Cholesterol
- High blood pressure
- Fatty Liver
- Sugar causes your skin to age by changing the collagen structure

- Fibromyalgia
- Heart Disease
- Cancer (Cancer cells are anaerobic – oxygen kills them. They FEED on sugar)
- Depression
- Mood Swings
- Irritability
- Anxiety or Panic Attacks
- Hyperactivity
- OCD (Obsessive Compulsive Disorder)
- Attention Deficit Disorder
- Learning Disorders, especially in children
- Anti-social Behavior (In studies, when delinquent children were put on a low sugar diet, a 44% decrease in anti-social behavior occurred)
- Anger Management Issues
- Aggression
- Neurotransmitter Deficiencies
- Insomnia
- Sleep very little
- Alcoholism

The American Diabetes Association considers consumption of refined sugar to be one of the three major causes of degenerative disease in America.

Simply NOT ADDING sugar to food and beverages yourself is not enough; you must diligently read labels and ask questions. Insure you know what is in the food and beverage you consume. Choose products that contain NO ADDED sugar OR the smallest amount of added sugar possible.

THE FDA
(OR Wolves in Sheep's Clothing and False Prophets)

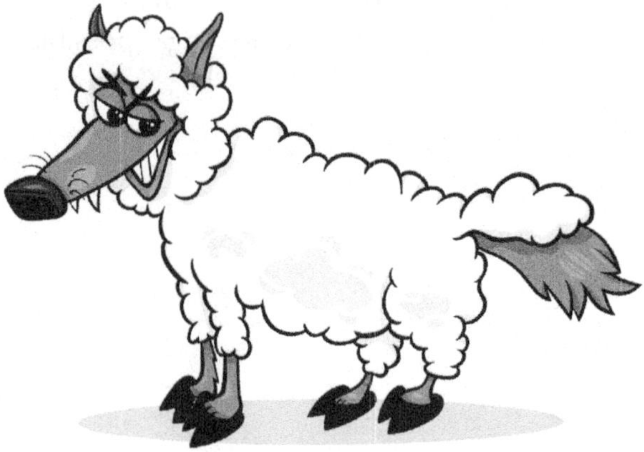

As you have been reading, you may be wondering . . . "Why the radio silence from the FDA? Aren't they supposed to protect us? What are they doing?"

The FDA is a government agency. They are ***supposedly*** an "unbiased" and "independent" government agency. Is any agency connected with Washington D.C. actually unbiased and independent? If you believe it is, I have a bridge I'd like to sell you.

Lead by and influenced by our government and (more to the point) the powerful lobbyists controlling our government, the FDA is ***SO*** concerned about the American public, it takes great pains to insure our food supply is raised using antibiotics, hormones, pesticides, and hundreds of other chemical substances in an effort to keep us (supposedly) "healthy." Due to the loving care lavished on us by the FDA, our food is pasteurized, homogenized, irradiated, gassed, engineered and genetically altered, absolutely guaranteeing that our food is stripped of vitamins, minerals, enzymes and most of its nutritional value.

If that's not enough, the FDA has been lobbying congress for decades to pass legislation allowing the FDA to control over-the-counter vitamins as if vitamins were prescription medication. The goal is to eliminate our access to vitamins and herbal supplements so that we are completely dependent on the medical community that is being paid NOT to help us (see Conspiracy Theory 101 for more information).

Don't think that by purchasing food labeled "organic" you will circumvent these practices and actually be bringing healthy food home. The FDA either allows or requires "organic" food to undergo these same processes with either NO labeling or minimal, vague labeling regarding what has been done to the food. Unless you are purchasing food that ***specifically details*** what procedures were ***NOT*** done to the food, you must assume the food has undergone every conceivable FDA approved process.

Remember when peaches were juicy, delicious and bruised if you laid a finger on them, and tomatoes were bursting with flavor but started rotting after only two or three days in the supermarket? You probably don't unless you are at least 40 or older. That's because peaches, tomatoes, and every other food we eat has been altered and engineered to insure it ***cannot*** be damaged in shipping and its shelf life will be extended as long as chemically possible so that profits are maximized. Everything is about the almighty dollar.

We all know that overeating is ***NOT*** the only reason people gain weight. If you didn't know it before, you should be crystal clear on this point by now. A malfunction of even the smallest organ can affect your entire body and cause obesity regardless of what you eat, or more to the point, do ***NOT*** eat. Similarly an imbalance in one part of your body may affect your entire system. For many (or even most) of us, obesity is ***merely a symptom*** of something systemic that has gone wrong.

One of the many problems with processed food is that the food is virtually devoid of enzymes. Enzymes affect our entire body and how our body digests and processes food. Enzymes are a critical component of the process of weight regulation. Food additives, preservatives and irradiation (all FDA approved) kill enzymes we need for proper digestion, processing food through our body systems, and weight regulation.

The FDA is fully aware that the requirements they allow and/or mandate destroy the nutritional value of food, and may even render some processed food hazardous to your health.

- Irradiation, for example, causes free radicals to form in the food, which may cause cancer. In the irradiation process not only are 5% to 80% of vitamins, minerals and enzymes stripped from food; cooking the food strips additional vitamins and nutrients faster and more comprehensively than cooking non-irradiated food.

- Antibiotics are passed from antibiotic treated food to us indiscriminately.
- Mad-cow disease is a man-made tragedy that occurred due to the FDA approved practice of grinding up the parts of domestic animals that were NOT utilized (bones, etc) and adding this disgusting stuff to the cow's FEED, thus making a gentle vegetarian animal a cannibal!
- Genetically altered food is so scary the imagination reels, and no long-term studies of the potential health consequences or horrors that may result from this practice even exist.

This is just the tip of the iceberg, yet the FDA marches forward with blinders firmly in place, ignoring danger, diseases, disabilities and deaths caused by their own requirements and approved practices.

Why?

Food, especially canned and frozen food, originally began to be mass-produced and distributed back in the 1940's and 1950's. People occasionally got sick, or more rarely died, because they ate a can of something that had a questionable seal, or they ate something that was past its expiration date. It's not as if this type of illness or even death was epidemic. Apparently the FDA would rather that we all died from the complications of poor nutrition, than have one idiot get sick because they ignored a bulging can top or an expiration date.

Most of the requirements mandated by the FDA are beneficial to (guess who?) the mega corporations that process, manufacture and distribute food. All of the FDA approved or mandated practices are primarily designed to make food more durable, resistant to shipping damage, extend shelf life, and eradicate pests such as fruit flies. It is also extremely important to recognize that many FDA requirements serve as a very high barrier to market entry for small companies that are not well financed, thus limiting competition. ***BUT***, what most people don't know is that the FDA's requirements don't cleanse, sanitize or sterilize food. In spite of all the processes food undergoes, if food is not stored and handled properly, bacteria can still easily thrive, making food toxic and people sick. So who exactly is the FDA protecting?

The FDA is a public regulatory agency with very broad powers. The ***stated*** mission of the FDA is to protect the citizens of this country from companies that, in the interest of their own corporate greed, would cause harm to the American people in the development, manufacture or distribution of drugs or food products. However, the FDA has become a Wolf in Sheep's Clothing that has been corrupted and has morphed into the role of safeguarding and increasing the profit margins of these mega-corporations regardless of the harm they do to us. Shockingly, in spite of scandal after scandal rocking the FDA for almost as many decades as the FDA has existed, most people are completely unaware of the FDA's duplicity.

On August 1st, 2005 a Wall Street Journal headline report indicted the FDA for actively concealing for many years the fact that canned tuna contained levels of mercury ***exceeding*** the FDA's **own** published "safe" mercury levels ***by more than 50% to 60%!*** The FDA ***NOT ONLY*** hid this fact, they ***admitted*** they placed canned tuna on their list of mercury safe foods in order to protect the profitability of the very lucrative, politically powerful, food industry, especially the extremely profitable canned tuna industry!

It is well known that the FDA also conspired with the dental industry for decades, continuing to provide support and FDA approval for mercury amalgam fillings, even though the FDA was well aware that mercury amalgam fillings were poisoning us. If you still have mercury fillings in your teeth you should look into having them replaced.

Mercury in any amount is toxic to humans. Mercury can come from many sources environmentally, but few sources are as hazardous as ingestion. It is well known that many of the fish in our food supply contain mercury. This is because governments worldwide, including the U.S., continue to allow waterways and oceans to be contaminated by mega corporations dumping their toxic garbage.

But how much mercury is actually "safe" to ingest? The FDA's published standards were already as high as possible to protect both the food industry and the corporate polluters. That the FDA actually concealed for years the fact that canned tuna was basically toxic waste in a can, should have resulted in officials going to jail. But since the FDA's actions were carried out at the behest of the highest levels of the U.S. government, who were coerced by the politically powerful food industry, no one was blamed for this mind-boggling event which resulted in untold damage to the health of millions of people, especially children!

The tuna industry defended themselves by publishing internally done studies that claimed most U.S. individuals ate only 10 cans of tuna a year. Really? Is anyone really so naïve they are fooled by such self-serving statements?

Although obesity is not among the symptoms normally listed in connection with mercury poisoning, mercury toxicity can result in an inability to lose weight. Mercury is among the toxins the body cannot break down and rid itself of without help. Consequently, if mercury (or other toxins of this type) is present in your body, in order to protect your brain and other body systems from continuous damage, the body will do what it can to limit the damage by storing these toxins in fat. Your body will also then create a very high level of resistance to releasing the fat, since release of the fat will release the toxic substance into your body and your organs.

Mercury damages the neural system and the endocrine (thyroid and adrenal) system most dramatically, but causes damage to many other parts of your body as well. So even ***IF*** you solve a thyroid and adrenal issue, if you still have mercury toxicity, you may continue to have a significant problem losing weight.

One of the most frightening aspects of ingesting too much mercury, especially for children, are the learning disabilities, autism and other cognitive disorders caused by mercury.

Testing for mercury and heavy metal toxicity is fairly simple. If you test positive, the treatment for this type of toxicity is known as chelation. Chelation is a chemical process whereby a chemical that passes harmlessly through your body bonds with the toxin, causing the toxin to then pass harmlessly from your system together with the chelation agent. Chelation was originally developed as a treatment for lead poisoning, but is effective for treating toxicity of many heavy metals and other types of chemical toxicity. I highly recommend undergoing intravenous chelation as that is the quickest and most comprehensive method. But oral chelation is available as well and is more convenient for some people.

Another unbelievably egregious action of the FDA occurred on March 22, 1990 when the FDA banned consumer sales of L-tryptophan in the United States.

L-tryptophan is an amino acid that humans and many mammals ***REQUIRE*** to be healthy. But L-tryptophan cannot be produced by the body on its own, so it must be gained via diet or dietary supplement. L-tryptophan is necessary to the production and regulation of

- serotonin (which prevents and relieves depression, as well as reducing pain sensitivity, anxiety, stress, PMS and assists in weight regulation),
- melatonin (which was detailed in the chapter on Sleep and Circadian rhythm)
- Lactic acid (which is the main catalyst for muscle repair, muscle regrowth, and is involved with endorphin production and mood regulation).

L-tryptophan is naturally present in many foods, but some foods are especially rich in L-tryptophan including turkey, milk, black walnuts, almonds, sesame seeds, pumpkin seeds, tofu and others.

Prior to the FDA ban, L-tryptophan had been sold for decades as a dietary supplement, and was even utilized by the medical profession to relieve depression, anxiety, PMS, control pain, promote natural sleep, and sometimes in treatments for alcoholism.

L-tryptophan supplements have *NO KNOWN NEGATIVE SIDE EFFECTS*.

In October of 1989 a batch of L-tryptophan that was ***contaminated*** due to manufacturing process error was shipped to the United States from Showa Denko, a Japanese company. The contaminated L-tryptophan was implicated in an outbreak of a rare disease called Esoinophilia-Myalgia Syndrome ("EMS") which includes symptoms such as severe muscle and joint pain, high fever, swelling and shortness of breath. There were approximately 1,500 total cases of illness with 38 fatalities attributed to the contaminated batch of L-tryptophan.

While there is no doubt this situation was tragic, there have been thousands of instances of contamination of pharmaceuticals and foods, including Tylenol (several independent incidents), Perrier, Rolaids, Benadryl, Lipitor, toothpaste poisoned by antifreeze shipped from China, and literally thousands of others, ALL of which resulted in widespread illness and/or death without the culprit products being banned by the FDA.

In the case of L-tryptophan, on March 26, 1990, the FDA banned all sales of L-tryptophan in the United States.

Just ***FOUR DAYS*** later, on March 26, 1990, Newsweek Magazine featured a cover article praising Eli Lilly's drug, Prozac, a relatively new, very expensive anti-depressant.

Prozac, (Fluoxitine, fluoxetine hydrochloride) also interacts with serotonin but ***VERY DIFFERENTLY*** from L-tryptophan. Prozac does ***NOT*** cause our body to produce or regulate serotonin. Prozac is one of a class of pharmaceuticals known as Selective Serotonin Reuptake Inhibitors (I dare you to say that five times real fast), which supposedly enhances the effects of serotonin our body has already produced, although the literature on how Prozac works in our body is so mysterious it can only be understood by rocket scientists.

In contrast to L-tryptophan supplements which (again) have ***NEVER HAD ANY KNOWN*** negative side effects, Prozac has a pages-long list of very frightening side effects which affect 4% to 20% of treated patients. ***A FEW of the KNOWN*** side effects of Prozac include psychosis, paranoia, delusions, depersonalization syndrome, abnormal dreams, anxiety, bizarre behavior, severe mental or mood changes, aggressiveness, hostility, hallucinations, irrational behavior, seizures, **homicidal actions, and suicide**. And this is the drug the FDA approved for treatment of depression?

By 1992 the FDA had reports of over 28,600 adverse reactions to Prozac, and an additional 1,700 deaths had been attributed to Prozac. So why didn't the FDA ban Prozac? Maybe these statistics got lost among the approximate 100,000 deaths that are attributed ***EVERY YEAR*** to FDA approved pharmaceuticals.

David Kessler, who was Commissioner of the FDA from 1990 to 1997, in an interview about the problems with Prozac stated, "Although the FDA receives many adverse event reports, these probably represent only a fraction of the serious adverse events encountered by providers. Only about one percent of the serious events are reported to the FDA, according to one study." So by inference, Commissioner Kessler was admitting there could have been over 2.8 million unreported adverse reactions to Prozac by 1992.

Since many domestic farm animals ***DIE*** if they do ***NOT*** receive L-tryptophan supplements in their food, the FDA allowed L-tryptophan to continue to be distributed as bulk-feed additives for commercial farmers raising cows, hogs, and chickens. L-tryptophan was also available to veterinarians caring for pets and horses. Apparently the importance of the health of human beings ranked below chickens, hogs, cows, horses, and household pets in the view of the FDA.

L-tryptophan was never banned in any other country, and was widely available in health food stores for people in many countries ***outside*** the U.S. such as Canada, the Netherlands, England, Asia, etc.

To add insult to injury, on February 9th, 1993, US government patent #5185157 was issued allowing **L-tryptophan** to be used as a **treatment and cure for EMS**; the very same condition that the FDA originally claimed was caused by L-tryptophan resulting in the ban on sales. The FDA also allowed L-tryptophan to be sold as a ***prescription drug*** only under a doctor's order at a cost of $75.00 for 100 capsules. The same 100 capsules had previously cost approximately $15.00 in health food stores prior to the sales ban.

What was formerly called EMS is now called Fibromyalgia. Obviously, since the FDA **claimed** the cause of EMS was L-tryptophan, it would be impossible for the same disease to appear in patients with no access to L-tryptophan. So a new name was needed, even though the symptoms are . . . wait for it . . . ***IDENTICAL!***

Eli Lilly's patent on Prozac expired in 2001. It is very illuminating that within a year after the patent expired the FDA quietly lifted their ban, once again allowing consumer sales of L-tryptophan for human consumption. All of this makes it painfully clear that the FDA conspired with Eli Lilly to guarantee that the pharmaceutical giant pocketed billions in profits from Prozac as well as its other drugs in the same genre, Zoloft and Paxil. The FDA graciously banned L-tryptophan, thereby eliminating the competition Eli Lilly faced from a benign, cheap, proven, safe, effective and natural dietary supplement.

Imagine the heartburn of a pharmaceutical company that has spent hundreds of millions or billions of dollars developing a new drug, only to find that patients prefer cheap, over-the-counter dietary supplements which do a better job of treating the problem and are far healthier. But (damn the luck) those pesky natural substances can't be patented!!!

The FDA is right there staunchly supporting the pharmaceutical giants and having sympathetic labor pains. On June 15, 1993, the FDA's Dietary Supplement Task Force published a report which stated on page two: "The Task Force considered various issues in its deliberations; including . . . ***what steps are necessary to INSURE that the existence of dietary supplements on the market does NOT act as a DISINCENTIVE for drug development.***"

It seems the FDA has found a way to provide the assistance the pharmaceutical industry needs. I imagine all the people who had adverse reactions to Prozac and other prescription drugs (especially the people who died and their families), wish the FDA cared a little less about the profit margin of the pharmaceutical industry and cared a little more about the people the FDA is ***SUPPOSED*** to be protecting.

The FDA has so clearly been corrupted by the money and political power wielded by the pharmaceutical and food industries, it is remarkable that the agency continues to exist. From bribery to favoritism to misuse of power the FDA does it all over and over again. If the C-level officers of most corporations did even one of the things the officials of the FDA have done, they would surely be in prison.

The FDA has vigorously and egregiously tried to gain control over "Dietary Supplements" (vitamins, minerals, and herbal products sold in health food stores) for decades. If this were to ever happen, you can be sure that we would find ourselves paying for doctor visits to get prescriptions for vitamins, and paying ridiculous prices at pharmacies for supplements that currently cost very little and keep us healthy.

In the early 1990s, the FDA publically declared "dangerous" many supplements commonly used and moved to ban them from consumer sales including CoQ10, selenium, chromium, and others. The American public's revolt against the FDA's ridiculous assertions resulted in the passage of the Dietary Supplement Health and Education Act (DSHEA) in 1994. This Act defines dietary supplements (including naturally occurring vitamins, minerals, herbs, botanicals and amino acids) as FOOD and not drugs, which is legally critical to the American public having unfettered access to high-quality natural supplements. The act also spells out regulations for the manufacture and sale of dietary supplements, and gives the FDA regulatory authority over dietary supplements within the context of the Act.

Don't think for a minute the DSHEA has stopped the FDA's campaign to limit our access to low-cost, natural, substances. As recently as 2010, the FDA had legislation proposed that would have eviscerated the DSHEA and eliminated our ability to walk into a Health Food Store and decide for ourselves what vitamins and other dietary supplements we want to take. The 2010 bill, with the deceitful misnomer "Dietary Supplement Safety Act of 2010" did **NOT** pass, thank goodness!

Our doctors and the AMA are willing participants cooperating with and encouraging the FDA in their efforts to eliminate our access to these products, because our access to vitamins and other natural dietary supplements with which we can keep ourselves healthy takes revenues and income away from doctors. Most of my doctors laugh at me for taking vitamins, constantly telling me that vitamins don't do anything except make my pee very expensive.

The FDA is working hand in glove with big corporate pharmaceutical and food industry interests as well as the medical community to deceive and rob the American public at the expense of our health. There is no telling where this will stop, if it ever does.

This chapter gives an extremely limited overview of just a couple of examples of things the FDA has done that show their true colors. The information presented above is only a ***very tiny sample*** of how the FDA's actions negatively affect us on a continuous basis, specifically concentrating on actions of the FDA that have ***DEFINITIVELY*** contributed to the obesity problem, and the difficulty many of us face in our attempt to control our weight. There are so many examples of the FDA's malfeasance that it would take shelves and shelves of books to cover it all.

Numerous books and tens of thousands of pages of documented evidence of the FDA's corrupt and reprehensible actions have been written by experts with far more credentials than I have in this area. In fact, my "credentials" on this subject are limited primarily to being smart enough to research and read thousands of pages of documents published by experts in this field. If you want additional information, you don't have to go any farther than the internet to find more books, documents, and articles than you can read in a year. Visit our website for links to information regarding more of the FDA's antics.

CONSPIRACY THEORY 101: *(CORPORATE AMERICA, INSURANCE COMPANIES, AND THE U.S. GOVERNMENT CO-CONSPIRATORS IN A LONG-TERM CON TO SUBVERT OUR HEALTHCARE AND OUR HEALTH)*

Younger people today don't even know what healthcare used to be like in the United States, back when we all had actual control of our own healthcare, our own doctors and our medical insurance. Prior to 1985 (give or take a year or two):

- Everyone chose their ***OWN*** doctor (no, not from a list published by an insurance company; you went to ***ANY DOCTOR*** you wanted to see).
- When something was wrong, you saw any doctor or specialist you thought might be able to diagnose the problem or help you. ***You didn't need anyone's permission.***
- Your doctor prescribed the treatment(s) or medication(s) the ***DOCTOR BELIEVED*** would best address and cure your medical issue. Your doctor was not required to follow procedures set out by the FDA to diagnose or treat your issues (procedures that fail 20% to 40% of all patients),

and neither you nor your doctor had to get permission from anyone before the doctor ***prescribed the best treatment(s) or medication(s) FOR YOU***.

- You were responsible for paying the doctor. However, most doctors and hospitals were either paid directly by the insurance company OR agreed to wait for payment until ***after*** you had received the insurance reimbursement.
- Then you or your doctor/hospital submitted the bill to your medical insurance company for the insurance reimbursement.
- Under the terms of most medical insurance plans back then, you were reimbursed approximately 80% (more or less) of the amount you had paid out, regardless of whether you had paid $10 or $10,000.
- If you didn't think a doctor was prescribing the appropriate treatment, you got a second opinion, or switched doctors. ***It was up to you!*** Your medical insurance company was required by law to pay for second and even third opinions.
- No one – absolutely no one – had any right to any information about your health, your medical conditions, or your health care. ***Especially NOT your employer***. It was the law!

Wow, imagine that! Radical Stuff!! A right to actual privacy AND to get whatever treatment or prescriptions you and your doctor agreed were the best options for you.

Then as now, approximately 50% of people who HAD medical insurance got their medical insurance through their employer as part of their Employment Benefits Package. Approximately 15% of the US Population was uninsured then; now, under Obamacare, approximately 10% of the US Population is still uninsured. However today, medical insurance premiums have increased to many times their cost in 1985 – since 2014 alone most medical insurance premiums have more than doubled, and deductibles have gone up so dramatically many people never even MEET their deductible anymore and are never actually reimbursed for anything!

Back then everyone knew doctors were generally well off, many of them still are. But they deserved to be, didn't they? They spent years in school – very expensive schools. And yes, doctor visits were more expensive than most of us liked, and paying out all that money and waiting (sometimes weeks) for the reimbursement check from our insurance company could be a hardship. But the system worked pretty well.

Yes, there was that 15% of the U.S. population that did not have medical insurance then. But these people could always get treatment if anything were really wrong – all they had to do was go to an emergency room or a free clinic. This was America, and our medical system was known for being one of the best in the world. People came from all over the world to see doctors, and to have surgeries here.

Back then, for all the people who got their medical insurance from their employer as part of their benefits package, most of them made a whopping contribution of about $50.00 monthly toward their medical insurance, whether they were single, married, or had a family.

Then Corporate America woke up.

Long before the 1980s, for several decades in fact, Corporate America had been following a practice known as "self insuring." The corporation would do a risk assessment, and "insure" themselves. This means that rather than pay big premiums to the insurance company, for certain types of insurance the company would take the lion's share of the risk themselves (usually up to a certain amount, say $500,000 or $1 Million), and then buy a very cheap "catastrophic coverage" policy (with a deductible in the amount the company was covering themselves), in the event there was a "catastrophically" large claim.

Originally companies started out with easy to assess risks such as auto insurance for corporate owned vehicles and rental cars (did you know the ***average*** claim for an auto accident is only approximately $2,000?). Then gradually, over the next couple of decades, companies began to "self-insure" almost everything for which they would have previously purchased insurance. This resulted in bigger profits for the Corporation, because if they "self-insured" wisely, they didn't have to pay out all the huge premiums required for full insurance coverage. Less expense for the Corporation means higher profits for the Corporation and more money in the bank for the Corporation.

Eventually the corporate bean counters began looking longingly at employee medical insurance. It was a huge expense for the Corporation, but the risk factors were incredibly difficult to calculate, and the bean counters didn't have any information to make an assessment ***because they were barred by law from invading the private medical records of their employees***, which were (frustratingly) sitting right over at the Insurance Company. Insurance that Corporate America was paying for! What to do, what to do? This intolerable situation had to be resolved.

In order to make a substantive change in the situation, something radical was required. Doctors usually practiced alone, or in small groups, so they didn't have any power to threaten the Corporation's machinations. The employees were a problem though. They were loyal to their doctors, and they had all these pesky legal rights to privacy and unfettered access to medical care.

In Board Rooms across America, the problem was under intense scrutiny. High priced consultants worked feverishly, plans were made. All powerful Corporate America would not tolerate the situation any longer; there was too much money at stake.

Then the first salvo was unleashed. Suddenly, out of the blue, there was a firestorm in the media (which was, of course, mostly owned and controlled by Corporate America) accusing doctors everywhere of deceiving and bilking their patients. According to the media, doctors were guilty of routinely running unnecessary tests, prescribing unnecessary medications, and even doing unnecessary surgeries just to enrich themselves!! How awful! Wealthy doctors taking advantage of their unsuspecting, trusting, patients and doing harmful things to them just to make a few additional dollars, when the doctors were already far better off financially than most of their patients. It was offensive! It was outrageous!

It was (mostly) a ***BIG FAT LIE*** told to a gullible public who believed anything they read in a newspaper or heard on CNN.

Who were these smarmy doctors? Does anybody know? Not really. One or two doctors may have been prosecuted very publically for things they may not even have done. But ***MOST*** doctors, who were caught actually committing ***any*** crime, were over-billing or double-billing Medicare. Committing insurance fraud may harm the insurance companies, or the tax payers. But it certainly wasn't what the doctors were being accused of. ***HOWEVER***, the important agenda of Corporate America was to divide and conquer – separate the patients from their doctors – and for that, the patients' faith in their doctors had to be destroyed.

Corporate America started rolling out their plan as slyly as a pride of lions hunting zebras.

It is important to remember that doctors aren't psychic and medical diagnosis and treatment is not a precise science. Even today, with all the miraculous advances in medicine since 1985, the diagnosis process is still mostly educated guesswork. The treatment that works for these nine people over here, may not work for the tenth person. And there is no way to make the process exact until we can manufacture human beings to exact specifications. But of course, this bothersome detail was never mentioned in the media firestorm – if the media had thrown in this small detail, it would have been counter productive to the power play Corporate America had put in motion. The media's job was to viciously slander and vilify doctors, and scare the public to death.

What is an unnecessary test anyway? If the results of a test are negative, does it follow that the test was unnecessary? ***Emphatically NO!*** The results of the test ruled out something the doctor suspected could be an issue based on the symptoms. A negative test result helps a doctor focus and narrow the diagnosis process. If a woman you love has a lump in her breast, do you want the doctor guessing whether or not the lump is benign? Or do you want the definitive results of a test showing a positive or (hopefully) negative result?

Now the stage was set, Corporate America and the Insurance Companies rolled out their plan.

HMOs were born.

Patients (employees) were co-opted to accept the new medical insurance structure by presenting the patients (employees) with the very attractive option of seeing a doctor and *ONLY* making a small "co-payment" at the point of service. For people who were used to paying out of pocket and waiting weeks or months for reimbursement from the Insurance Company, this seemed like a *VERY* attractive option. Now the patient (employee) didn't need to worry about the actual cost of the doctor, prescription, test or hospital visit – the patient (employee) does what they need to do, and all they pay is a small co-pay. The Insurance Company (and, unbeknownst to the employee, ***their employer***) take care of the rest! And under these new insurance plans the experts at the Medical Insurance Company would be watching over the greedy doctors to make sure they were only running tests the patients actually needed, prescribing the "right" medications and generally doing what the Insurance Company (and Corporate America) told the doctor was best for the patient.

Corporate America embraced this new plan.

Then the downside began to kick in. Suddenly people found they had fewer choices than before – they now had to choose their doctors from a small list of "participating" doctors. But hey, this new medical insurance plan was still pretty good, no more out-of-pocket-costs, and one doctor was surely as good as another, right? And the media said the savings would be huge! This new structure was going to lower the cost of medical care AND the cost of medical insurance for everyone.

Now the Insurance Company (quietly fronting for the Wizard of Corporate America behind the curtain) had a firm stranglehold on the doctor's livelihood. Doctors were always the most vulnerable link in the chain, ***because*** they practiced individually or in small groups, and back then hospitals tended to be stand alone organizations or small groups of hospitals might be jointly controlled. But now the Insurance Company (who was fronting for their boss, Corporate America) had control of the patients, who could ***ONLY*** see doctors on the Insurance Company's "List."

To have a practice (and a continued livelihood), it was imperative that the doctor be on the Insurance Company's almighty "List."

Most doctors are just like us, they have families and mortgages and bills to be paid. To stay in business in the new world of HMOs and Managed Care Insurance Plans they ***HAD TO*** accept insurance, otherwise most of their patients can't afford to see them. Under the new insurance plan structures, many plans ***only*** allow insured participants to see "In Network" doctors. Even plans that allow participants to choose "Out of Network" doctors make sure that seeing an "Out of Network" doctor is financially onerous so participants are strongly incentivized to see the "In Network" doctors the Insurance Company (and Corporate America) has the most control over.

Suddenly doctors were being told by Insurance Companies that Procedure A should only cost $40.00, Procedure B should only cost $25.00 and a standard office visit could only cost $XX.00; amounts that were a reduction of 50%

to 80% of what the doctor had previously been charging patients.

Many people believe each doctor elects which insurance they will accept. That used to be true, before 1980 or 1985. Today the opposite is generally the unfortunate reality. Doctors negotiate the best contract they can with one or two insurance providers and the patients now under the control of those one or two insurance companies become the vast majority of the doctor's business.

Being expelled from Insurance Company's plan would be the death knell of most doctors' practices – especially when ***ALL*** the Insurance Companies are offering virtually identical basic packages to the doctor and have set up virtually identical prices for services the doctors are ***allowed*** by the Insurance Companies to offer to patients.

Resistance was futile. Most doctors had no choice but to knuckle under to the tyrannical coup d'état of the newly created dictatorship, regardless of how they felt about the situation ethically or morally. Then when Obamacare came into being, the insurance company regulation of the doctors became even more onerous.

Today virtually ***ALL*** medical insurance plans have some very fundamental things in common. Things many people are completely unaware of:

- Most large corporations are "self-insured" for the medical insurance of their employees. (Large corporations still account for nearly 50% of all people who have medical insurance.) Small companies that have so many employees that they are actually required to offer medical insurance, typically purchase medical insurance policies for small businesses through an insurance company. 37% of people are covered by the government primarily under Medicare or Medicaid. The other approximate 7% of people who HAVE medical insurance coverage, purchase individual policies through their choice of medical insurance providers (or, now, through the Affordable Care Act portal).

- When a Corporate Employer is "self-insured" the employees are typically unaware of this fact. The Corporation pays an Insurance Company a small annual fee to "administer" (or front) the insurance plan, make the rules (at the Corporation's direction), process the claims, and negotiate with the medical providers, such as doctors, hospitals, pharmaceutical companies, etc. The Corporation pays into an internal corporate account established for this purpose all the "Medical Insurance Premiums" collected from their employees and the matching funds contributed by the Corporation. From this account, the Corporation pays an "Administration Fee" to the Insurance Company, AND the Corporation reimburses the Insurance Company dollar for dollar for all monies paid out in claims. Any "profits" in the internal Corporate Account (monies that are not paid out to the Insurance Company) are kept by the Corporation. The goal is (of course) for the Corporation to make a profit on the medical insurance of their employees. This also results in an extra added incentive for the Corporation to make sure that their workforce is young and healthy, and thus requires less medical care.

- Insurance Companies (in cooperation with their client, Corporate America), have structured contracts with participating medical providers (doctors, hospitals, pharmaceutical companies, etc.) so that:
    - Doctors are ***PAID BONUSES*** to ***REFRAIN*** from running tests on patients, especially expensive tests. If a doctor runs too many tests, funds due to them from the Insurance Company may be forfeit, or the doctor may be ***expelled*** from the insurance plan completely.
    - Doctors are ***PAID BONUSES*** to ***REFRAIN*** from referring patients to specialists. If a doctor refers too many patients to specialists, funds due to them from the Insurance Company may be forfeit, or the doctor may be ***expelled*** from the insurance plan completely.
    - Doctors are ***PAID BONUSES*** to ***ONLY*** prescribe the particular medications that are listed in the Insurance Company's "Formulary". (A "Formulary" is a listing of specific medications "preferred" by the insurance company.) Doctors who prescribe *NON*-Formulary medications face reductions in payments or non-payment of monies due them, OR the doctor may be ***expelled*** from the insurance plan completely.
    - Insurance Companies are paid "Revenue Sharing" by pharmaceutical companies ("Revenue Sharing" is a politically correct term for contractual kickbacks) to induce the

Insurance Company to add medications manufactured by the pharmaceutical company to the "Formulary" of the Insurance Company. Arrangements where the Insurance Company agrees to exclusively list in their Formulary a single specific medication for a certain condition results in higher revenue sharing payments than non-exclusive arrangements. The more medication purchased by patients insured under the plan, the greater the "Revenue Sharing" payment from the pharmaceutical to the Medical Insurance Company (a pro-rata part of this payment is obviously passed on to the Corporate Client of the Insurance Company). It is an interesting fact that it is illegal for a doctor to receive kick-backs from a pharmaceutical company, but it is NOT illegal for an insurance company.

- Some insurance plans pay doctors a set fee per patient, and it is up to the doctor to work within the amount of money paid to them by the insurance company when providing treatment to each patient. If the doctor spends additional time and resources on a particular patient, making that patient's care more costly, the doctor makes less money; OR if the patient needs too much care, it could actually cost the doctor money to treat the patient effectively. If you believe doctors who work under this type of arrangement with the insurance company actually provide the highest standard of care to their patients, I have a bridge I'd like to sell you.

- In many medical insurance plans even ***IF*** a doctor wants to prescribe tests, treatments or specialist consultations for a patient, these types of services must be pre-approved by the insurance company before the services may be prescribed or rendered. The result is that accounting clerks are second guessing our doctors and deciding what care the patient may or may not have.
    - Since the beginning of HMOs, insurance Companies have published lists of standard procedures and protocols to be utilized in diagnosing and treating most illnesses or conditions – the more common the condition, the stricter the standards. These lists set out the diagnostic procedures, tests, protocols, and treatments doctors within the insurance company's "Network" are ***authorized*** to utilize to diagnose and treat patients. Unsurprisingly the allowed procedures and protocols usually include the cheapest choices that could be made, which aren't necessarily the BEST choices, and certainly aren't usually the most up to date choices for diagnosing and treating your medical issues. If doctors frequently go outside the Insurance Company's guidelines they are subject to expulsion from the Insurance Company's Network. Since the advent of Obamacare, the government has gotten involved in institutionalizing these types of standards and protocols – the government feels that if the standards in place work for 80% of patients they are good standards. The 20% of people these standards do not work for? Well,

they will just have to get along without appropriate medical care.

- When doctors sign contracts with Medical Insurance Companies to become part of the "Network" of the Insurance Company, the contracts contain "confidentiality" clauses legally ***BARRING*** the doctor from disclosing the terms of the contract, ***especially*** from disclosing how the doctor is compensated (or bribed) by the Insurance Company. So even ***IF*** the doctor ***WANTED*** to tell you that they are being coerced and bribed by the Insurance Company to provide sub-standard care to you, the Insurance Company (backed by your employer and/or the government) could sue the doctor for disclosing confidential information and ***you*** could likely sue the doctor for malpractice. So doctors have a **huge** vested interest in claiming they are doing the right thing for you and it is coincidental that they are paid extra money by the Insurance Company for the recommendations and treatments they have provided to you at the behest of the Insurance Company (and Corporate America and the United States Government).

- Many Insurance Companies retain the contractual right to unilaterally amend the terms of their contracts with doctors, including the right to amend lists of acceptable clinical protocols and procedures, without any notification to doctors or any ability on the part of the doctors to prevent such changes. So even well meaning, ethical, compassionate doctors who want to do the right thing can be baited and switched by an Insurance Company (working in cooperation with Corporate America and the US Government) and literally be contractually prevented from giving you healthcare the doctor believes you need.

- Insurance Companies pay hospitals within their Networks substantial bonuses to ***REFRAIN*** from exceeding target levels for many services (meaning the hospitals must withhold such services from most patients) including services such as emergency services, tests, treatments and specialist referrals.
- The fine print of most medical insurance policies today gives the Insurance Company co-ownership of patient medical records. The Insurance Company can then legally use those records however they want, even if the use is detrimental to your interest. And the Insurance Company has a contract with your Corporate Employer and/or the US Government granting access to your medical records to your Employer and/or the US Government. Your Employer and the US Government now has continuous detailed insight into your health and any conditions you may have.
- Under many insurance plans, doctors are held to specific maximum targets with regard to hospitalization, specialist utilization and emergency room utilization. The doctors are financially rewarded for coming in below maximum targets, the further below, the greater the reward. If they EXCEED their maximum target they may be

subject to financial "disincentives" (meaning the doctor forfeits money they would otherwise have been paid by the Insurance Company) or expulsion from the Insurance Company's Network.

It is obvious that the best doctors to see are doctors that do ***NOT*** participate in any HMO or Insurance Company Networks. However, these "Rock Star" doctors who are so sought after that people will pay anything to see them, regardless of whether or not the Insurance Company will reimburse, are both expensive (as they are generally at the top of their field) and very difficult or impossible to get an appointment with because they are in such demand.

Unfortunately most of us can't afford to pay out of pocket for the services of these Rock Star doctors and then PRAY we receive some level, however pitiful, of reimbursement from our insurance provider (which will usually only reimburse the approximate $45.00 the Insurance Company would have paid a doctor participating in their Network – the standard office visit reimbursement MINUS the co-pay you would have paid at one of their participating doctors).

I am old enough to remember when you could see any doctor you wanted and, as long as your reason for seeing the doctor was valid; your Insurance Company reimbursed 80% of the cost.

Corporate America and the Insurance Companies coerced ("lobbied") the cooperation of the U.S. Government to make the decision that regulating the medical field as if it were a public utility is constitutional (it isn't), proper (it's not) and beneficial (to whom?). Under the brave new world of modern medical insurance plans and Obamacare, most doctors are paid identical fees for service under the contract terms "negotiated" (or dictated) by the Insurance Company, regardless of the doctor's qualifications, background, or expertise. Ditto hospitals, labs, specialists and other medical service providers.

You think this a good thing? Really? Would you buy a car if the government forced the car manufacturer to cap the cost of safety features at an 80% reduction from yesterday's price? And the car manufacturer now has to recover their cost, pay their employees AND show a profit on the safety features. What do you suppose would happen to the quality of the auto's safety features? Scary thought?

Where in our capitalist society did it get written that doctors are a public utility and that all of them should be paid equally, regardless of their qualifications, their experience, or how good they are as a doctor? Or that an accounting clerk should be allowed to dictate to a doctor how they are required to conduct our medical care?

When these changes occurred, the cost doctors paid for office rent, overhead, staff, insurance, etc. was their own problem, and of course these costs varied based on the area where the doctors practiced. For the doctors their costs hadn't changed and still had to be paid. So doctors were forced to see exponentially more patients or be put out of business.

Suddenly the quiet reception area at my doctor's office, where I used to pass a peaceful 20 minutes while I waited with two or three other patients to see the doctor, was now a mob-scene where I waited for 2 hours with 30 or 40 other patients to spend 2 minutes with a doctor who was now forced to see 4 or 5 times the number of patients they saw previously just to maintain their income.

In the early years, premiums were a little bit lower for the new HMO and Network types of "healthcare" plans. But in just a few years premiums reached levels amounting to many times what medical insurance had previously cost – and, lo and behold, some self-insured corporations were now making substantial profits on the insurance premiums. To add icing to the cake, Corporate America suddenly found themselves in an employer's market and started passing more and more of the "cost" of the medical insurance premiums to their employees.

Less than 3 years after the company I worked for in 1985 converted to one of the new types of medical insurance plans, the $50.00 per month I had for many years been contributing to the cost of my medical insurance as a single person became a whopping $150.00 per month, then continued to rise to over $350.00 per month. I was ALSO faced with the disconcerting fact that NONE of my doctors were in the new insurance plan "Network", so I had to switch to new doctors, or pay out of my own pocket for my medical care and receive virtually ZERO reimbursement. Today, under Obamacare, medical insurance premiums have skyrocketed, and according to analysts will only continue to rise.

Every time there is public discussion of ***the rising cost of medical INSURANCE***, the Insurance Companies simply cite ***rising medical COSTS*** and go on about their business.

Today all we hear all the time is that doctors charge too much and medical costs are out of control. But many people don't realize or understand that the doctor's *"PUBLISHED"* fee schedule is actually a work of fiction. No one really pays those amounts for the doctor's services, unless they have *NO* medical insurance whatsoever. (And people who have no insurance probably aren't seeing the same doctor you see.) In reality, the doctor is being paid whatever pittance the Insurance

Company has decided is the ***"normal"*** fee for each service the doctor provides and the doctor is forced to run a business and pay themselves a salary from that severely reduced amount.

A doctor who has a "published" fee per office visit of $200.00 is likely only receiving approximately $60.00 per office visit under the guidelines of their contract with the Insurance Company. No one has any idea how much doctors (and hospitals and other medical service providers) would actually charge for their services if they were not forced to artificially inflate their published fees for ALL services as a negotiating tactic with the Insurance Companies.

It is mysterious why people don't seem to realize that medical costs have been artificially inflated BY the very actions of Corporate America in cahoots with the Insurance Companies, and then exacerbated by the US Government under the Obamacare laws.

When you hear or read about "rising healthcare costs," the prices cited are the artificial retail price tags, it's irrelevant whether the price tag cited is a doctor office visit or a hospital stay. The cost cited appears astronomical and frightening. It is designed to make people ***WITH*** medical insurance grateful to their employer and/or the US Government for the insurance.

Further, these types of statistics are designed to make the public at large feel sorry for folks, especially children, without medical insurance. Have you ever noticed that when politicians talk about people with no medical insurance, they play on people's heartstrings by trotting out stories about charming two year old toddlers that are gravely ill whose parents have no medical insurance because they have been laid off after decades dedicated to a single company? Why do these politicians rarely ever talk about the adults who don't have medical insurance because they refuse to work, are irresponsible, are illegal aliens, OR maybe they are under 30 and are simply taking a calculated risk they won't develop any chronic illness, or 100 other politically undesirable reasons an adult might not be purchasing medical insurance.

It is important to remember that the Insurance Company is ***ONLY*** paying their ***NEGOTIATED*** price for the item or service cited – and the negotiated price is a discount of 50% to 90% off the published retail price.

Healthcare costs are rising significantly ***PRIMARILY*** for uninsured individuals who actually have money. Those who are indigent receive free healthcare paid for by taxpayers. And now those same taxpayers are footing the bill for the insurance subsidies granted to a substantial percentage of the US population.

At the time of the initial changes in medical insurance structures, doctors I saw who generally charged $85.00 to $100.00 for an office visit found themselves under contract with the Insurance Company to receive about $40.00 for an office visit for any patient insured by the particular insurance plan. The $40.00 being the amount that the insurance company had determined through some magic formula was the correct amount for an office visit with a doctor of this type.

Doctors make HUGE investments in their careers. Why shouldn't they make a good living? The cost of medical school is hundreds of thousands of dollars over 4 years (which comes ***AFTER*** getting an undergraduate degree which took 4 years prior to starting medical school). ***THEN*** if the doctor is pursuing a specialty, there may be additional years of school. ***THEN*** doctors spend an additional 2 years being paid a pittance and abused with 100+ hour work weeks as residents.

Most doctors charge far less for their time than lawyers. Interesting that we don't see many headlines about the exorbitant cost of lawyers, and how poor children are unable to afford good legal services. Gee, do you suppose that's because lawyers create most of the laws and become politicians who pass the laws into existence? It is guaranteed that we will never see the day that a lawyer's income is capped or that there are headlines about the exorbitant cost of legal services.

Imagine the dilemma suffered by a young or middle-aged doctor. For the first time in history doctors today face income restrictions never contemplated by prior generations of doctors. The doctor has office costs, exorbitant costs of malpractice insurance, hundreds of thousands of dollars in student loan debt, and a family to support. Now imagine you are that doctor and you are forced (by the Insurance Company you absolutely cannot afford to alienate) to choose between ordering tests you believe a patient needs ***OR*** your child's orthodontia requirements which would be covered by the bonus the Insurance Company pays you for ***NOT*** running those tests.

Even the most benevolent, altruistic person would find themselves making Hobson's choice in this Occam's razor situation. For most of us, the scale would probably tip in favor of our family – and there you have it.

It has long been a truism that "you get what you pay for." It is pretty clear that Insurance Companies, Corporate America and the U.S. Government are willing to pay ***ONLY*** for sub-standard medical care for most of us.

There are thousands of cases of people whose health has been irreparably compromised or who suffered fatal consequences because they were denied medical tests, necessary treatments, or medications by their medical insurance provider. I myself know at least 8 or 10 people who have suffered permanently damaged health or who have died as a consequence of bean counters running the show. And I know dozens more people who had vicious battles with their medical insurance provider before they could get proper care.

And yet I've never known, or even heard of, one single specific person who was the victim of an unscrupulous doctor that ran unnecessary tests or performed unnecessary operations.

The sweeping changes in medical insurance that got us to where we are today was an enormous fraudulent scam perpetrated by Corporate America in collusion with insurance providers with the blessing of the corporate controlled U.S. Government. The result is that Corporate America, Insurance Companies and the U.S. Government have taken control of the medical industry. Corporate America and Insurance Companies are making a ***MUCH*** bigger profit on medical insurance and the medical industry in general, by putting the doctors under the thumb of Corporate America. It is clearly Corporate America who was the original driving force behind the curtain directing their mercenary henchmen, the insurance providers who now pull the purse strings on the puppet doctors, and now the US Government has joined the club.

Corporate America and insurance providers, as the master architects of these, so-called, "healthcare" insurance plans were (and still are) laughing up their sleeves all the way to the bank.

Meanwhile, all the senior corporate executives are cared for by extraordinarily expensive, high end institutions that specialize in and provide Executive Medical Care to Corporate America. The bill for this is footed, of course, courtesy of Corporate America, under the guise of a fiduciary obligation to make certain that their corporate executives are healthy and taking good care of their stockholder's money.

Have you noticed when change is gradual most people seem not to really notice or care? It is an interesting facet of human nature that people get comfortable with the status quo and they simply go with the flow. Even if the flow doesn't make them completely happy, it is what they have become used to, and it's easier than rocking the boat. The powers that be use this demonstrable human characteristic to their advantage constantly.

There were several class action lawsuits over these types of insurance plans, and the way doctors are now rewarded (bribed) by the insurance providers to work in opposition to the interest of their patients. The fact that these lawsuits were struck down on primarily technical grounds without a murmur from the media was a sure sign that the U.S. Government (at the direction of Corporate America) had decided the new order of corporate/government controlled healthcare and medical insurance was here to stay.

As they were institutionalized, these new types of medical insurance plans became more and more unassailable. Even the media (controlled, of course, by Corporate conglomerates and the US Government) allows themselves to be manipulated into the politically desirable supportive position on the issue. And of course since Obamacare came into being these insurance plans have become government sanctioned to the point that insurance plans that provide more flexibility are being virtually outlawed.

Medical insurance plans became more and more sophisticated under the guidance of corporate analysts, who slice and dice the mounting data (now that the Insurance Companies, Corporate America and the US Government have ownership of everyone's medical records) to determine how best to cost control the medical process.

Under the new strictures, even if people don't realize it, medical treatment is becoming more and more like an assembly line where each step is performed with robot-like precision to the most cost-effective (cheapest) specifications. "If patient has symptoms A and B, run test C – test D is not approved for use in this scenario." Anomalies that disrupt the assembly line cannot be tolerated, as they are costly. So patients that require more care, or whose conditions are difficult to diagnose are shunted to the sidelines more and more frequently.

It is interesting (and a little bit frightening) that when politicians want to do something that is likely to be unpopular, they give it a name like the "Patriot's Act." That way for those inconvenient nay sayers who have the temerity to point out that the "Patriot's Act" actually stripped away the rights of American Citizens to privacy and Due Process, all the politician needs to do is finger point and loudly as possible proclaim that the nay sayer is NOT A PATRIOT! Wow.

The so-called "Patient's Bill of Rights" is a fairy tale that was politically desirable to make everyone more emotionally comfortable without actually disrupting the new order, where doctors do what the accountants (directed by your employer and Uncle Sam) tell them to do (no matter what might have been best for you), and your medical history is being used against you. What rights? The doctors do what they are told and aren't allowed to even tell you they ***WANT*** to do something else or something different. The Insurance Company, your employer and the US Government (by contract with the insurance provider) co-own your medical records.

Patient's Rights are a fairy tale designed to make you believe you really are safe and sound, all little girls really do grow up to become princesses, and of course, everyone really does live happily ever after.

A similar myth is that generic medications are exactly the same as brand name medications. Of course they aren't. A $10.00 bottle of wine has the same basic ingredients as a $300.00 bottle of wine, but they sure don't taste the same. And the $10.00 bottle will likely leave you with a hangover, because of the cheap ingredients used to make it.

Generic medications are required by law to have the same basic active ingredients as the brand name medication, but not necessarily in the same amounts or the same proportions. The regulations governing generic medications:

- Allow a generic to deliver 80% to 125% of the Active Ingredient into your bloodstream vs. the strict adherence the brand name medication must maintain on active ingredients
- Require that inactive ingredients ONLY be "similar" to the brand name medication
- Require ONLY that generic medication have **"SIMILAR"** RESULTS to the brand name medication
- Requires that the package insert for the generic version of a drug, show the actual data for the BRAND NAME version of the drug. While in actuality, the data for the generic drug is usually different.

The FDA doesn't release these facts to the consumer public.

If I'm baking bread and I decide to use 20% less yeast than is called for by the recipe, and I decide to use saccharine rather than sugar – is the bread going to be exactly the same?

It may still be bread. It may even taste sort of like the original bread (maybe) but will it taste good? Will it even rise?

FURTHER, there is no ability for a consumer to control **WHICH** generic version of the medication my pharmacy is buying on any specific day, I could get 20% LESS active ingredient delivered to my bloodstream this month and 25% MORE next month. In fact, if I took a generic that delivered 20% less active ingredient last month, and I take a generic that delivers 25% more this month, that's a 45% variance!

Exactly the same? I don't think so!

Do some generics have good results? Yes, they do. Do all generics have the same result as the brand medication? Absolutely not. But how would you know, since your insurance plan probably doesn't allow the brand medication to begin with.

Yes, it is very easy to criticize big pharmaceutical companies over the cost of brand name medications. But even though it may cost only 5¢ per pill to manufacture a medication that retails for $10.00 per pill, the pharmaceutical company incurred hundreds of millions of dollars or even billions of dollars of cost to:

- Do the research and development on the drug (this phase alone may take years or decades of investment). For major drugs approved in the last decade, R&D costs have ranged from about $3.5 Billion to as much as $12 Billion.
- Do all the necessary clinical trials and testing
- Get FDA approval, which can easily cost between $1 Billion to $4 Billion

- Market the drug
- Provide free brand name drugs to patients who can't afford them (my then 79 year old mother was the beneficiary of such a program at AstraZeneca after her mastectomy due to breast cancer)
- And ship free drugs to third world countries where no one can afford them.

And the pharmaceutical company has only about 10 years to recover their investment before they are required to give the formula for the medication to their competitors and generics are allowed to flood the market.

Of course today there is the additional wrinkle that many insurance plans don't allow costly new medications (no matter ***HOW*** beneficial they are) to be added to their "Formulary" due to the expense. So, your doctor may not even tell you about a new more effective medication that has just entered the market for your condition, because they will be financially punished by the Insurance Company if they write a prescription for the new medication. You yourself may not even ***want*** the new medication since your insurance provider won't pay for it. So, for financial reasons, patients are often forced to continue on older medications that aren't as effective, but which are available in a cheap generic form.

There are articles published by experts indicating that pharmaceutical companies have changed their focus away from expensive research and development of new drugs and treatments aimed at ***curing*** diseases, and instead are now focused primarily on new drugs and treatments that merely ***relieve symptoms***. Reasons cited for this change of focus revolve around several factors:

- There are far greater profits in medications which are primarily for cosmetic or lifestyle enhancing purposes that are usually not even covered by medical insurance plans, such as Viagra, Botox, sclerotherapy, or cryoneuromodulation

- Billions spend on speculative R & D may never be recovered if no new medication/cure is ever found OR is discovered first by a competitor

- Experts indicate it is often faster and less expensive to develop drugs and treatments to relieve symptoms

- Eradicating a disease or condition renders all the medicines and treatments developed for that disease/condition and relief of its accompanying symptoms worthless and expendable. Imagine how many drugs and treatments would experience severely diminished necessity or even become useless if cancer were permanently eradicated tomorrow

- There is more profit over the long term in relief of symptoms, because if the underlying illness is never cured, the need for medication that relieves the symptoms will continue indefinitely. Thus a guaranteed income stream is born.

There is a very disturbing logic to these lines of reasoning from a business perspective, although it remains to be seen if there really is a clear shift in this direction on the part of big pharma. We may never actually know for sure. After all, if a cure is never found for cancer, is it because there is ***NOT*** one, or because no one really tried?

When talking about the long list of medications insurance providers decline to cover, it is interesting (or disturbing) that many insurance plans *deny coverage for diet medications*, ***even for morbidly obese patients***. Most of these insurance providers express the view that weight loss is cosmetic in nature. This is not only another instance of discrimination against people who are overweight or obese, which is morally and physically debilitating to those of us suffering from weight problems, it is very dangerous.

Insurance Companies will sometimes, in the most extreme cases of morbid obesity, agree to pay for gastric bypass or bariatric surgery, which is life-altering, irreversible, and causes a multitude of serious, detrimental side-effects and health consequences. But they won't cover the cost of diet pills before things have gotten to that point. Can someone please explain this to me?

Why are Insurance Companies, Corporate America and the U.S. Government sticking their heads in the sand and purposely ignoring the fact that obesity is now the #1 leading disease in America (and the world)? There is no other condition from which over 60% of the United States population suffers. And obesity leads to a long list of serious or fatal physical conditions including diabetes, cardiac disease, liver disease, circulatory disorders, heart attack, stroke, and death. And many of the leading causes of obesity, such as thyroid disorders and sleep disorders are likewise being ignored and undertreated.

To add insult to the litany of injuries catalogued in this chapter, because of the way they are evaluated and paid today, many doctors are ***refusing to accept or are turning away*** patients with chronic medical issues. Of the many types of medical issues which have turned these individuals into pariah patients, the most shocking, appalling and (sadly) prevalent is ***obesity!***

A decade or so ago information started to circulate quietly in the media (usually buried in the back pages of small local and regional publications) about doctors that were refusing to perform surgery on obese patients due to the increased risk, both during the surgical procedure and of post surgical complications.

Over the years Corporate America and Insurance Companies have become more sophisticated in spinning statistics and have further and more elaborately refined their guidelines requiring doctors to meet lower and lower goals in the amount of care given to patients. These refinements have resulted in Insurance Company Network contracts with physicians where the doctors receive greater financial rewards for achieving the lower and lower goals for patient care demanded of them. Any patient that requires more resources or more care negatively impacts the doctor's income and the Insurance Company's statistics.

Make no mistake, as we have shifted the burden of paying our doctor bills to our Insurance Companies (our Employers or the US Government); the doctors have naturally shifted their loyalty and their primary allegiance to the entities that control the doctor's income.

It has become so commonplace for doctors to turn away patients because the patient is overweight; the August 2011 issue of Glamour Magazine ran a reader poll asking if this practice was fair on the part of the doctors! A shocking 47% of readers responded that ***YES, this practice is fair and ethical!!*** I guess those were the 47% of Glamour Magazine readers who have no weight problems.

One doctor interviewed for the article ***freely admitted in print*** that patients who are overweight require more procedures and tests and this factor made it more likely the Insurance Company would expel the doctor from their plans!!!

The U.S. Government, State governments and local governments not only endorse this type of policy, they participate in it.

There are extremely beneficial medical tests and procedures that are actually being made illegal in many instances. One prime example is laboratory testing for Lyme Disease; Lyme Disease is a disease that can be easily cured if diagnosed early, but this is frequently mis-diagnosed and if not treated early can be devastating, permanently debilitating and sometimes fatal. If your home or your doctor's office where the test results are to be delivered is located in New York State it is actually illegal for any lab in the United States to run the Igenex Lyme panel tests, the Bartonella FISH, the Lyme IgG/IgM/IgA Screen, or the Lyme PCR-W Blood test for you. Some of these tests happen to be the best, most definitive tests for Lyme disease, but they are actually illegal in New York State. Yes, there is actually a law about this! The illogical reason generally given for the illegality of these particular tests is that the tests result in too many "false positives." The reality is that New York State doesn't want to admit to their residents or to tourists that there is an epidemic of Lyme Disease in the State of New York that has been going on for years or decades. Of course, Corporate America and their insurance provider henchmen are just as happy not to pay for the prescription medication and treatments for the Lyme Disease epidemic.

This is only one small example of a problem that is pervasive and is becoming more common as accountants and analysts take charge of our medical care.

These same analysts and accountants are the very people who evaluate the risk of lawsuits for things such as unacknowledged Lyme disease epidemics, automotive gas tanks that explode on impact, pajamas that combust in flame, all product liability lawsuits, and medical lawsuits. All of these types of lawsuits are viewed similarly by Corporate America, and the risk of liability is carefully weight against the cost of voluntarily correcting the problem. The types of factors which might be evaluated include things such as:

- What is the cost of addressing the problem (medically treating everyone, correcting the defective product, etc.)
- The chance of whether or not anyone will ever even figure out there is a problem or even identify the source of the problem is carefully weighed. Often the risk the source of a problem will ever even be discovered is quite low. For instance, if a gas tank explodes in an auto accident, how many people think first of a defective gas tank as the problem, especially when gas tanks often explode as an ancillary event?
- Another big factor that is considered is the fact that filing a lawsuit against a large corporate or government entity is very costly and many people either can't afford to or won't file suit in the first place due to the potentially enormous expense/investment involved for many years litigating against such an entity. Especially when people weigh in the chances of losing the lawsuit and the money they have personally invested.

- Analysts evaluate the number of people who might be harmed and weigh that number against the potential of even more costly class action lawsuits being filed.

These are the types of factors that are carefully considered when corporate or government entities decide whether (or not) to actually admit a problem exists – regardless of whether the problem is a defective product or an epidemic. Will the cost of admitting the problem exists and fixing it outweigh the potential cost ***IF*** there were ever a lawsuit? All too frequently the answer is that keeping people in the dark, and doing whatever is necessary to keep people in the dark, is cheaper than the liability which MAY exist, maybe.

The rising health care problems in the United States are a direct reflection of the practices and mindsets discussed in this chapter. Obesity being one of the most prevalent and visible results of these policies and practices.

And this is probably just the tip of the iceberg. The U.S. Government not only ***ENDORSES*** these practices, it is going to great lengths to ***INSTITUTIONALIZE*** them legally in its national healthcare program which every citizen is legally required to participate in. Look at all the lies we KNOW about that President Obama told the American public to get the Affordable Care Act passed!

To me, these things are unbelievably frightening.

WRAPPING IT ALL UP AND PUTTING ON THE BOW

I know there are parts of this book that read as if it was written by a conspiracy theorist. Just remember, ***ALL*** the factual information in this book, and much, much more like it, is easily verifiable; visit our website for links to an amazing amount of information. Check out the facts yourself on the internet. The conclusions I have drawn based on the facts are my own.

I have lived the Dynamic Dining Design food program. The program has been modified and refined many times over the years based on evolving nutritional research I have continuously done. As I ***ALWAYS*** knew the only thing holding me back from my perfect weight was unidentified, improperly diagnosed or improperly treated health problems.

Dynamic Dining Design will work for virtually anyone, as long as you are certain your health problems have been identified and you are receiving proper treatment. Especially thyroid disorders and sleep disorders.

As I said in the beginning, there is information about dieting and obesity in this book that no one has ever told you before. I am not making this stuff up, nor do I get psychic messages from Edgar Casey.

After three decades of dedicated research, I simply realized available information was interlinked in ways it had never previously been presented! Pulling together information from various, seemingly unrelated areas, but which all affect our bodies, a coherent picture began to form. Extrapolating the details of the underlying reality in relation to obesity and weight loss, the picture became crystal clear.

For me, the last pieces of the puzzle fell into place when I finally (after 30+ years) got on the right thyroid medication *AND* I was (after more than a decade) diagnosed with sleep apnea. Once these two things occurred, by sheer coincide virtually at the same time, I instantly began to lose weight without even trying. It was an epiphany. Like a thunderbolt out of a clear blue sky, everything I learned over the decades of research, fell into place and made sense. I had to share what I know.

I can understand that someone might have read or might know all the same facts I have gathered over the years, and still not draw the same conclusions. But I find it surprising when I talk to people, especially those who have the same types of weight problems I do, who say they have never heard of many of the things I have read repeatedly for years, even things that were front page news – canned tuna, front page Wall Street Journal . . . never heard of it? How does that happen?

It's true, there is a lot of very confusing, false, and misleading information out there – put out by (guess who?) the medical community, the FDA and Corporate America (with the blessing of the almighty U.S. government).

Maybe everyone is struggling with memory issues from thyroid malfunctions, sleep deprivation and mercury poisoning. Or is it too tired from their sleep disorders. Or is it too beaten and insecure from years of emotional abuse by the medical community. Goodness knows I was!!

FOR DECADES I KNEW MY WEIGHT HAD NOTHING TO DO WITH WHAT I ATE. I also knew that there was nothing wrong with eating meat, and olive oil and eggs. It became very clear to me decades ago that our bodies were meant to process and run on abundant natural food sources – preferably *UN*-irradiated ones. But I had literally given up. I was beaten.

I had actually consciously decided there was nothing I could do anymore except eat the way I was eating. I knew I was eating healthy. I knew, regardless of anything anyone said, that what I weighed had absolutely nothing to do with what I put in my mouth. I ***KNEW*** beyond a shadow of a doubt that any ten other people, who ***DIDN'T*** have whatever mysterious problem(s) were causing my weight gain, and who ate what I ate, would be thin! I knew this in my soul so clearly it was irrevocable and steadfast. And yet, doctors never helped me – they simply kept repeating the same tired old clichés, chose to believe I was lying about what I ate, and refused to look beyond those two incorrect beliefs to help me or try to actually diagnose what was wrong. No matter what I did, or how little I ate, I kept gaining weight, and nobody would do anything to help me.

So I just gave up. After forty plus years, I wasn't going to fight it anymore; I was just going to be fat. I was done. And when I died young from diabetes, and cardiac problems and whatever, well tough – that's life.

Yes, there was a tiny little part of me that still cried out that I wanted to be pretty, and wear pretty clothes again. But I decided that was obviously never going to happen. I wasn't going to torture myself or beat myself up anymore. I was just done.

I guess hope springs eternal and I apparently still harbored a shred of hope I didn't even know was there. Because I did go to see this one new doctor who changed my thyroid medication, and sent me to this colleague who prescribed a sleep study. I still shudder to think what would have happened if I had said no.

After I was diagnosed with sleep apnea and I had that ***AH HA*** moment in the doctor's office, and then the weight kept coming off steadily even though I was eating exactly the same as before (or even eating more than before), I knew I had to do whatever I could to spread the word.

For myself, I desperately wish I had snapped in that last piece of the puzzle sooner. Here I am, past my prime and losing weight again for the first time in more years than I want to count. I wish I could have back all those years when I could have been wearing pretty clothes and feeling good about myself. Oh well. At least I was one of the lucky ones; I have a husband who loves me, whatever my weight, so I always felt loved. And now I can spend the next 30 years or so enjoying how I look and feel.

It is no accident that obesity is the number one leading disease affecting the U.S. population. Whether by accident or whether by design, the current overwhelming statistics on obesity are a direct result of the actions of Corporate America, Insurance Companies, the FDA, the U.S. government, and can be laid at the feet of the medical community who has done nothing to prevent it or to help. Rather than feeling beaten by our weight and the ancillary health problems that arise from obesity, all of us should be furious!

Here's something else the powers that be **won't** tell you:

IN ORDER TO LOSE WEIGHT, you must first UNDERSTAND and be able to EFFECTIVELY COMBAT ALL the factors AFFECTING YOUR WEIGHT and YOUR BODY'S ABILITY TO REGULATE YOUR WEIGHT

Since many of the factors preventing you from losing weight are ***CREATED*** by the very organizations who are supposed to be responsible for helping us and caring for our health, it is obviously ***NOT*** in their best interest to tell anyone anything helpful or give us the tools to effectively combat anything, is it?

It's nice that medical organizations wring their institutional hands over the "Obesity Problem." It would be even nicer if they stopped lying to us, or actually did something helpful.

Yeah, let's not strain our imagination.

The government regularly publishes propaganda about how unhealthy it is to supersize your Happy Meal. It's not just coincidental that this type of propaganda resulted in the ability of the Fast Food Industry to create new lines of "Healthy Alternative Cuisine" that isn't' really much healthier, but that resulted in billions of dollars of additional revenue for their restaurants. Amazing how that works, isn't it?

As long as all of these collective institutions and agencies keep falling back on the myth that ***"Calories In vs.***

Calories Out equals your weight," millions of people will needlessly continue to be obese.

- The actions and policies of the FDA are dangerous and certainly not in the best interest of the American people, especially those of us who are overweight. The FDA is bought and paid for by the pharmaceutical and food industries. The policies of the FDA, whether supported by or dictated by our government, insure that your body will, at the very least, have a grueling uphill battle losing weight (if you can lose weight at all), ***EVEN*** if you have ***ZERO*** medical problems.

- The medical community will continue to stick its collective head in the sand (or in other less savory dark places), ignoring the problem, refusing to treat those of us with weight problems, or even exacerbating the problems, ***UNTIL*** they actually see benefit in their financial bottom line by solving the problem through correct diagnosis.

- The pharmaceutical industry will continue to use their political and financial clout to keep everyone in the dark and obese until it's more financially rewarding to the pharmaceutical industry for people to be thin than it is for people to be obese. What? You don't think all of the profits pouring into pharmaceutical companies because of obesity and the numerous health problems resulting from obesity are lucrative for the pharmaceutical industry? Even ***IF*** they come up with a magic pill that makes people thin, it's a crap-shoot whether or not they will decide to market it – Yes, there have been estimates that such a pill would be worth hundreds of billions of dollars – But all the medications and treatments they sell now which are, at best, temporary "fixes" for obesity (which either never actually goes away OR comes right back), are worth hundreds of billions of never ending dollars from suckers like you and me who will buy anything that promises to make us thin. ***AND*** the medications and treatments sold for chronic conditions related to obesity, such as diabetes, cardiac conditions, and the numerous other health problems that arise from obesity, are also worth hundreds of billions of dollars. Make people thin, and all that money goes away. Need I say more?

Even ***IF*** there ever ***IS*** a magic thin pill, it will no doubt cause some new cancer or other equally devastating disease that will also require a cure, thus insuring the future of the well-lined coffers of the pharmaceutical industry.

- The government – well, they are going to go along with whoever has the deepest pockets, the most power, or best lobbyists (who have both money and power). The government certainly isn't concerned about you or me and our weight problems. We are nameless, faceless masses who aren't good for anything except a vote.

In the meantime, ***ALL*** of these factions want us to believe their myths. ***ALL*** of them.

It is past time to break free of the shackles of believing that Corporate America and the U.S. Government have our best interest at heart. They don't. And believing they do might kill you.

- Corporate America's #1 goal is to sell their products. In order to do that, there must be a need for their products. If there is ***NOT*** one, or if the need is not great enough to be satisfactory, they will not hesitate to ***CREATE*** a need.
    - Antivirus companies hire hackers to create and release computer viruses so that we are afraid to leave our computers unprotected. Are there real hackers trying to break into the Federal Reserve? You bettcha. But do you really believe anyone actually cares about the peach cobbler recipe Aunt Sally finally e-mailed to you? Or the few hundred dollars in your checking account? Seriously? Fortunately the Federal Reserve doesn't use the same antivirus software you and I use either, because if they did we'd all be in trouble.
    - Companies that used to be proud of the decades their products lasted now have "planned obsolescence." You needn't worry about the Maytag repairman; he isn't lonely or bored anymore. When you buy a TV today you know it won't last 20 years or more like the first TV your parents or grandparents bought back in the 1950's or 1960's. In fact, a lot of those old TVs are still going strong today; only thing is you can't get but 4 channels on them – and that's in small towns where there are still broadcast

TV signals and there is no interference with the rabbit ear antenna – since those TVs weren't cable ready! Today when you purchase a TV the salesman is upfront that the active life of the TV (or the washing machine, or the lawn mower or whatever) will be 7 or 8 years, assuming technology doesn't change and make the TV obsolete before then. Every electronic item we buy today is "planned" by the manufacturer to have a certain length of useful life, after which it breaks and must be replaced. Can you bend the odds by taking particularly good care of an item? Sure. But will it last forever? Absolutely not.

    - Companies that manufacture mousetraps probably have a secret mouse breeding program somewhere in the outback.

- The pharmaceutical industry is part of Corporate America, a big part. They too want you to buy their products. If you buy a 10¢ absolutely natural vitamin that makes you well and makes you feel ***BETTER*** than the $10.00 artificial chemical pill with 100 side effects the pharmaceutical industry would ***PREFER*** you took, it pisses them off. ***AND*** the FDA takes care to insure that the pharmaceutical industry is fat and happy. No matter what it takes.

- The medical insurance industry and your corporate employer want to make a profit on your medical insurance. They don't give a diddly damn about your health, as long as you can't definitively blame them for anything.

- And the government, ah, our ubiquitous government. Money and power . . . VS. Nameless, faceless, masses. Who do you think they care about?

It's your body and your health. You MUST take charge and become your own healthcare/medical advocate.

You can begin again.

- Start the Dynamic Dining Design program tomorrow.
- Keep your food journal.
- Find a doctor who will actually help, who is willing to take the time and run the tests to diagnose the health problems you ***KNOW*** or ***SUSPECT*** you have that are preventing your body from properly regulating your weight.

Dynamic Dining Design can result in your very own magic "thin" genes. Stop eating rice cakes and plastic food and eat like a normal person again. Food is good for you. It's supposed to taste good, too.

Know that you are ***NOT crazy***. There ***IS*** something wrong if you can't lose weight, and there ***IS*** help. Check out our website, visit often for updates, the latest information and resources.

Today is the beginning of a beautiful, new, **THIN** you!

APPENDIX #1: VITAMINS

It is important that you take vitamins, both for your overall health, as well as to promote your body's ability to properly regulate your weight.

The food we eat (whether fresh food you are lovingly preparing, or processed food you are quickly zapping) has been rendered virtually void of vitamins, minerals and essential nutrients. It has been engineered, picked unripened, gassed, irradiated, homogenized, pasteurized, and processed to the point that so much nutritional value has been stripped it's a wonder people are even able to walk around.

It's not enough that FDA required and approved practices strip our food of virtually all nutritional value. At the behest of the Pharmaceutical Industry (that not so secretly calls the shots at the FDA) the FDA has repeatedly tried to take control of all vitamins and natural supplements so that it can make the wet dream of Big Pharma come true by removing vitamins and natural supplements from the consumer market.

Denying the American Public access to vitamins and supplements that keep us healthy, would protect Big Pharma's onerously expensive, chemically engineered, side effect laden pharmaceuticals from competition by cheap, healthy, natural substances, and at the same time tickle the fancy of the AMA by forcing you to pay for a doctor visit every time you wanted a prescription for a (now egregiously over-priced) jar of vitamins.

Virtually no one has died or even had a serious adverse reaction to natural vitamins and supplements during the last century. The FDA has the unequivocal authority to pull from the market any "supplement" that illegally contains prescription or banned substances.

YET, the FDA has repeatedly had legislation proposed that would ban consumer access to healthy, natural vitamins and supplements completely or make them all prescription only.

Every time the FDA has colluded with some legislator who is controlled by the pharmaceutical lobby and actually gotten legislation proposed, it is always egregiously disguised to deceive both congress and the public into believing that the legislation actually has our best interest at heart. Fortunately, the latest example of this type of flagrantly dishonest legislation (with the duplicitous misnomer "Dietary Supplement Safety Act of 2010") did ***NOT*** pass. Thank goodness!

Every U.S. citizen, regardless of their weight or their diet, should be taking vitamins and supplements.

Not all doctors are fans of nutricuticals. In fact, your doctor may laugh at you, or even actively advocate that you do ***NOT*** take vitamins. ***Ignore them***. Vitamins never hurt anyone. Vitamins can ***ONLY*** help you, even if your doctor doesn't agree.

It is virtually impossible to overdose on most vitamins. The government RDA is barely enough of most vitamins to keep you alive, so you should generally take at ***LEAST*** 2 to 4 times the daily RDA of any vitamin.

Many books and some doctors advocate taking vitamins as often as 4 to 6 times a day. This is too labor intensive for me. If I try to get that detailed, I end up ditching my vitamin routine. I would suggest that you take vitamins 2 times a day – before breakfast and after dinner. Vitamins generally absorb into our system most effectively if taken close to a meal when you have food in your system. Tryptophan in particular needs to be taken at dinner time or even later, about an hour before bedtime.

Just as a "CYA" I am going to advocate that you consult with your physician before beginning any vitamin regimen.

DAILY VITAMINS/SUPPLEMENTS RECOMMENDED

VITAMIN/ SUPPLEMENT	Highly Bio Available Form	MINIMUM Acceptable	MINIMUM Recommended	OPTIMUM DOSAGE
Vitamin A	Micellized Vitamin A	2,000 IU	3,500 IU	8,000+ IU
Thiamine (B1)	Liposomal Vitamin B Complex	10 mg	25 mg	50 mg
Riboflavin (B2)		10 mg	25 mg	50 mg
Niacin (B3)		15 mg	40 mg	80 mg
Calcium Pantothenate (B5)		25 mg	50 mg	100 mg
Pyroxidine HCI (B6)		10 mg	25 mg	50 mg
Biotin		100 mcg	300 mcg	500 mcg
Folic Acid		400 mcg	600 mcg	800 mcg
Pantothenic Acid		50 mg	100 mg	250 mg
Vitamin B12		200 mcg	400 mcg	800 mcg
Vitamin C	Liposomal	1,000 mg	2,000 mg	3,000+ mg
Vitamin D3	Micellized Vitamin D3	400 IU	800 IU	1,000+ IU
Vitamin E	Micellized	200 IU	600 IU	1,000+ IU

	Vitamin E			
Calcium	Calcium Orotate	1,000 mg	1,500 mg	2,000 mg
Magnesium	Magnesium Chloride	100 mg	200 mg	400 mg
Potassium		100 mg	200 mg	500 mg
PABA		50 mg	100 mg	250 mg
Chromium Picolonate	Sublingual	120 cg	100 mcg	250 mcg
Choline		25 mg	50 mg	100 mg
Pantethine		100 mg	200 mg	400 mg
Natural Sea Kelp Iodine	Liquid	100 mg	200 mg	400 mg
DHEA	Liposomal	25 mg	100 mg	200 mg
Lethicin		50 mg	200 mg	500 mg
R-Alpha-Lipolic Acid	Liposomal R-Alpha-Lipolic Acid	25 mg	50 mg	100 mg
CoQ10	Liposomal	30 mg	100 mg	500 mg
Essential Fatty Acids (Omega 3, 6, &9)		500 mg	1,000 mg	2,000mg
Multi Amino Acid		1,000 mg	2,000 mg	5,000 mg
5 HTP		25 mg	50 mg	100 mg
CLA		50 mg	100 mg	500 mg
Digestive Enzymes		Read packaging and dose as recommended		
Pro-biotics (General)		Read packaging and dose as recommended		
Lactobacillus Gasseri		1 Billion CFU	2 Billion CFU	3 Billion+ CFU
Lactobacillus Plantarum		1 Billion viable organisms	5 Billion viable organisms	10 Billion viable organisms
L-Glutathione		10 mg	50 mg	100 mg
L- Glutamine		25 mg	50 mg	200 mg
L-Carnitine		25 mg	200 mg	500 mg
L-Tryptophan (At night before bed)		25 mg	500 mg	1,000 mg
Fiber		Both Insoluble (such as Chia Seeds) AND		

		Soluble Fiber should be taken. Read packaging and dose as recommended		
Ultra Greens		Read packaging and dose as recommended		
Citrus bioflavonids		100 mg	500 mg	1,000 mg
Grapefruit Extract		Read packaging and dose as recommended		
Olive Leaf Extract		Read packaging and dose as recommended		
Zinc (Chelate)		25 mg	50 mg	150 mg
Selenium		70 mcg	200 mcg	500 mcg
Copper (Sulfate)		1 mg	2 mg	2 mg
Manganese (Chelate)		5 mg	5 mg	5mg
Luetin		25 mg	50 mg	200 mg
N-Acetyl Cysteine (NAC)		25 mg	50 mg	200 mg
Lyopene		25 mg	150 mg	100 mg
Quercitin		25 mg	50 mg	100 mg

APPENDIX #2: TIGHTENING UP AS YOU LOSE WEIGHT

In addition to regular exercise, if you were more than 30 pounds over your optimum weight when you started the Dynamic Dining Design program, you may find that tightening up and toning your body is essential. Toning exercises should be done in ***ADDITION*** to your regular exercise.

It is best to start toning activities early in the weight loss process, and keep at it as you lose weight. The toning process does not need to be an onerous activity, nor does it need to take up much time.

There are a few very easy "exercises" here that can be done by virtually anyone, regardless of how overweight or out of shape.

These "exercises" are targeted to tone and tighten those areas that are generally the most problematic areas. Even if you do ALL of these activities morning and night, it should not take more than 30 minutes (total) out of your day.

Many thanks to my niece Miranda Fegan for the illustrations in this Appendix.

TUMMY TONER

Lie flat on your back on a carpeted floor, yoga mat, your bed (if it is not too soft), or any other firm surface that will support you without interfering with the exercise.

Cross your arms over your chest

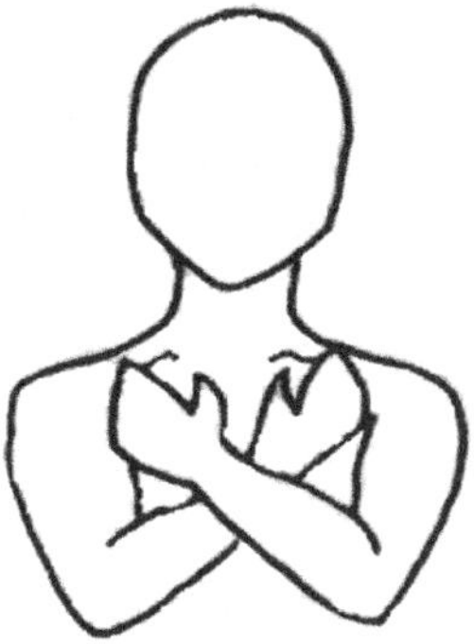

Raise your shoulders and your legs simultaneously approximately 4 to 6 inches off the surface and hold for a count of 10.

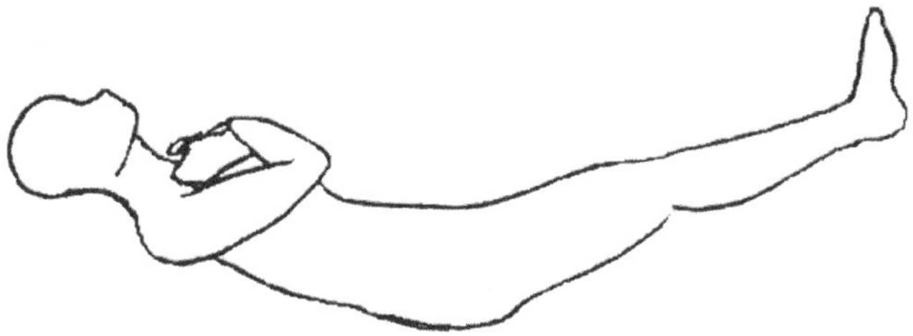

Repeat 10 times.

BUTT & THIGH TONING

Lie on your back with your knees bent and pressed together.

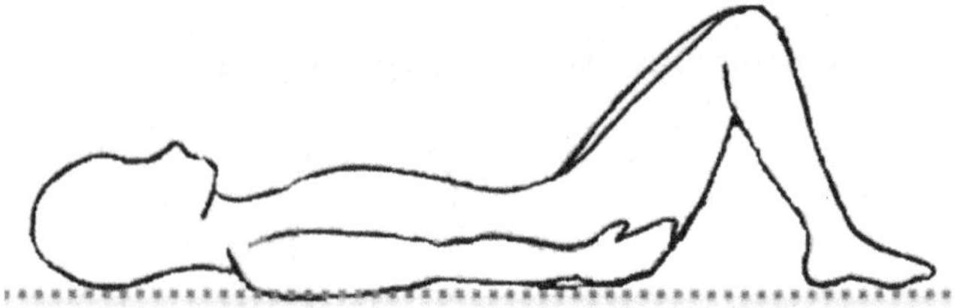

Lift hips off the floor as high as you can.

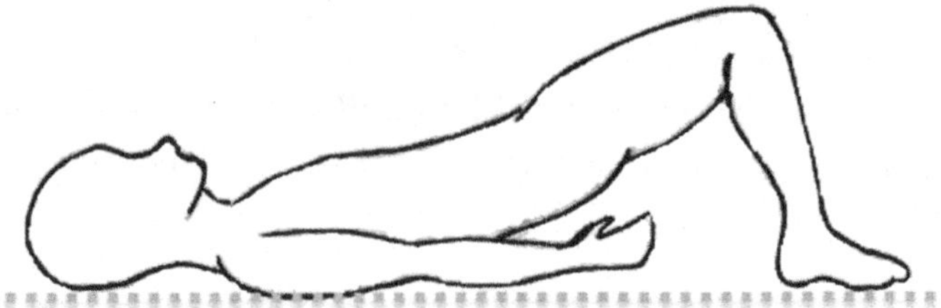

Repeat 10 times.

Spread knees shoulder width apart and repeat 10 more times.

THE CHAIR

(Targeting Butt & Thighs)

This is easy to do while on the phone, if your phone is near a wall or on the wall (or wireless or mobile).

Stand with your back flat against the wall. Your feet spread shoulder width apart and approximately 12 to 16 inches in front of you.

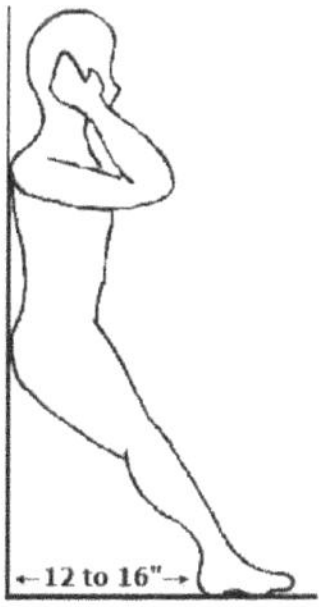

Slowly slide down the wall until you are in a position as if you are sitting in a chair.

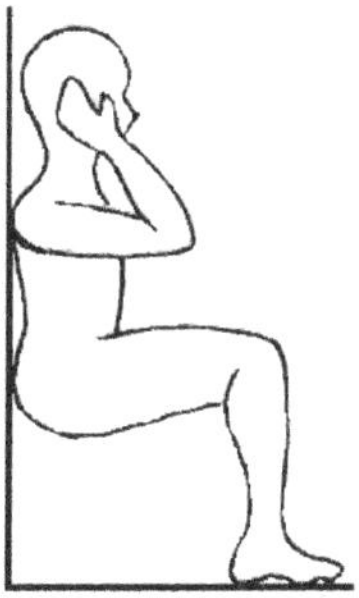

Hold 10 seconds (or as long as you can) and slide back up the wall. Repeat as many times as practical.

LOVE HANDLE ELIMINATOR

This will get rid of those annoying bulges on the sides of waist.

Stand with your feet apart a little more than shoulder width. Your arms straight out on both sides at shoulder height.

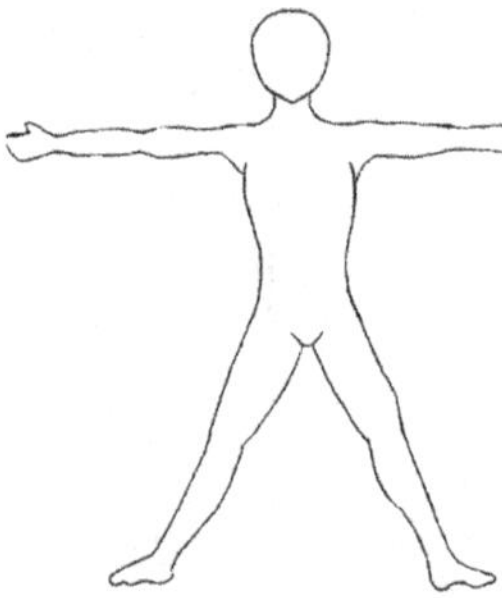

Bend to the right – let your right arm reach toward the floor and your left arm curve naturally over your head so you feel the stretch in your left side.

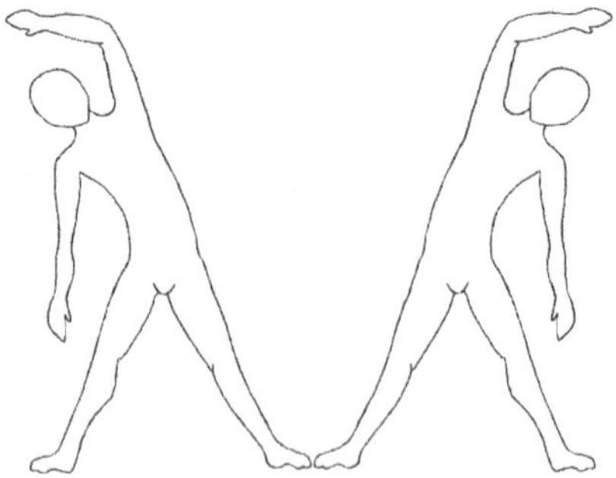

Repeat 10 to 20 times on EACH side of your body.

SAGGY ARM STRIKE DOWN

Stand with your feet approximately shoulder width apart and your arms out to the side at shoulder height.

Make little circles with your entire arm. 10 to the front, 10 to the back.

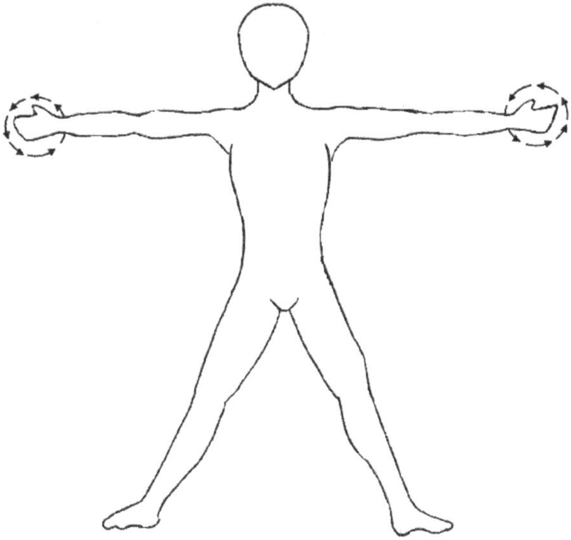

Repeat 5 to 10 sets.

FOR THE TA-TAs

Nothing has ever equaled the power of the oldie, but goodie – the isometric exercise designed to tighten saggy pectoral muscles.

Whether standing or sitting up straight, put your palms together right over your pecs and press palms together until you feel the tightening in your pecs. Do this over and over while repeating after me.

"We must, we must, we must increase the bust…"

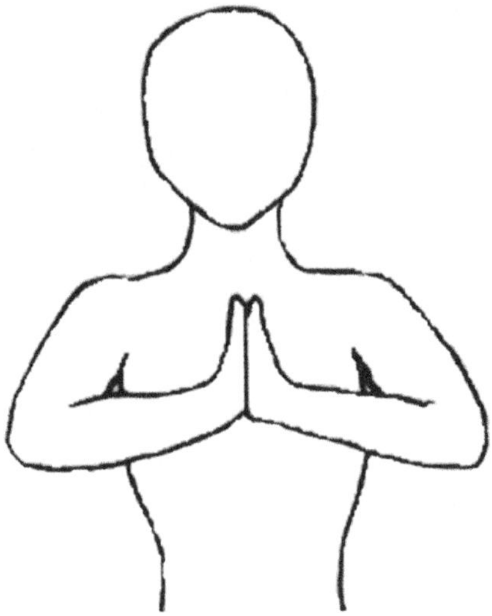

APPENDIX #3: FOOD LABELS

Reading and understanding food labels is critical. This cannot be stressed enough. *NEVER* purchase anything that actually has a food label without ***reading*** the label. All food labels are required by U.S. law to include specific information, much of which is very helpful to everyone following the ***Dynamic Dining Design*** program.

- Be CERTAIN you understand what the label designates as a *"SERVING SIZE"*. Many times I have purchased an item thinking the container held one serving and that the calories and carbohydrates listed on the label were reasonable for a single serving. *ONLY* to get home and look at the label again and discover that the company believes there are *FOUR* servings in there. For who? Toddlers? When viewed as 4 times the calories and carbohydrates, the item suddenly becomes *MUCH* less appealing.

- All nutritional information given on the label, such as the number of calories, the number of carbohydrates, etc. should be broken down on a *PER SERVING* basis. This is why it is vital to make sure you find the serving size and understand how many servings are in the container.

- The most important information on the label is generally:

- Calorie Count
- Carbohydrate Count
- Sugar Grams
- Sodium (if that matters to you)

INGREDIENTS: TOMATO PUREE (WATER, TOMATO PASTE), DICED TOMATOES, HIGH FRUCTOSE CORN SYRUP, MODIFIED FOOD STARCH, ONIONS, SALT, CORN STARCH, ONION POWER, DEHYDRATED GARLIC, SPICE, CITRIC ACID, BASIL FLAVORING, ASCORBIC ACID (ADDED TO HELP RETAIN COLOR), MILK, MONOSODIUM GLUTENATE.

Nutrition Facts

Serving Size 1/2 Cup (114 Grams)
Servings Per Container 2.5

Amount Per Serving	
Calories 100 Calories from Fat 10	
	% Daily Value*
Total Fat 1g	**1%**
Saturated Fat 0g	**0%**
Polyunsaturated Fat 1g	**1%**
Trans Fat 0g	
Cholesterol 0mg	**0%**
Sodium 820mg	**34%**
Total Carbohydrate 23g	**8%**
Dietary Fiber 2g	**8%**
Sugars 16g	**0%**
Protein 2g	

Vitamin A	15%	Calcium	4%
Vitamin C	30%	Iron	6%

*Percent Daily Values are based on a 2,000 calorie diet. Your Daily Values may be higher or lower depending on your calorie needs.

	Calories	2000	2500
Total Fat	Less than	65g	80g
Sat Fat	Less than	20g	25g
Cholesterol	Less than	300mg	300mg
Sodium	Less than	2,400m	2,400mg
Total Carbohydrate		300g	375g
Dietary Fiber		25g	30g

- It is critical to pay attention to the amount of sugar and to understand whether any sugar contained in the product is **NATURALLY OCCURRING** sugar that is inherently part of the natural food (for instance, corn, whether picked fresh in a field, canned, or frozen, naturally contains approximately 1 gram of sugar per 8 oz cup of kernels), ***OR*** if some form of processed sugar has been ***ADDED*** to the food. Especially in processed foods. If a product contains ADDED sugar I try to find a similar product that does NOT contain added sugar. But, if even 1 gram of sugar is listed on the nutrition label, ***READ*** the ingredients carefully. ***ADDED*** sugar is found in the most unlikely foods and is cleverly hidden in the list of ingredients utilizing terms you may not recognize as sugar. Some of the names utilized for added sugar that may appear in the ingredients list are:

- High Fructose Corn Syrup (HFCS)
- Fructose
- Dextrose
- Maltose
- Lactose
- Sucrose
- Anything ending in the letters –ose
- Sorbitol
- Mannitol
- Hexitols
- Barley Malt
- Brown Rice Syrup

- Molasses
- Honey
- Date Sugar
- Maple Sugar
- Turbinado Sugar
- Agave
- Organic Cane Syrup
- Fruit Juice

BEWARE! The list above may not be comprehensive. The food industry constantly makes up **new** names for added sugar so that consumers don't realize sugar has been added.

Added sugar is so insidious; there are even brands of SALT that include added sugar!

Even if you have been buying a product for years and think you know what is in there, it's a good idea to check the label every few months. Companies change formulas and ingredients all the time and you may find that added sugar has made its way in there – just like I discovered it in my Tomato Soup.

APPENDIX #4: BODY MASS INDEX (BMI)

Calculating your personal Body Mass Index (BMI) is a somewhat overrated activity. Personally, I can just look in the mirror and know whether I am fat or not.

In recent years some parts of the medical community have also started to question the value of BMI calculations. After all, if your BMI is 25 or 26, are you really unhealthily overweight? Probably not. But I can tell you without question, if your BMI is over 40 or over 50 or even higher (like mine was), there's no question you are in the extremely unhealthy overweight category. But then you can probably look in the mirror and know that without doing the math.

BODY MASS INDEX (BMI) CALCULATION

$$\frac{\text{Your Weight (In Pounds) x 703}}{\text{Your Height (In Inches)}^2} \text{ (Divided by)}$$

So, to calculate my BMI when I weighed 274 pounds, the calculation was:

My weight 274 (lbs) multiplied by 703 = 191,922

My height 64 (inches) multiplied by 64 (inches) = 4,096

191,922 divided by 4,096 = 46.8 (or 47 rounded) BMI

Yep, I was pretty unhealthy. But I could see that in the mirror, and I could tell by the fact that if I walked more than one block I was out of breath. I wore a size 26 for pete's sake, that's a hint.

BODY MASS INDEX (BMI) RANGES

18.5 – 24.9	Healthy
25.0 – 29.9	Overweight
30.0 +	Clinically Obese

This will give you some idea what your doctor may be thinking from a medical perspective, and may help you determine what a more healthy weight is for you. If your BMI is 26, and you feel good and look good, I wouldn't sweat it. But if you feel better and look better at a weight that puts your BMI at 21, go for it. It's a personal thing, and medical science is starting to admit that the chart above is not meant to be rigorously adhered to by everyone.

APPENDIX #5: TYPICAL MENUS & MEAL SUGGESTIONS

In the following pages you will find examples of typical meals. For those who prefer structure and limited choices, 10 days of menus have been provided until you get the hang of the Dynamic Dining Design program. Creative mixing and matching will result in limitless days of menus if desired.

Mix and match the breakfast, lunch and dinner menus as you wish. Don't forget snacks – eating the two daily snacks at appropriate intervals between meals will help keep your blood sugar level and help you get through the day without being hungry.

You should ***NEVER*** be hungry on the Dynamic Dining Design program. Do your best to establish a reasonable dining schedule (within the parameters of your life) and do your best to stick to it; following this guideline should preclude excessive hunger at any point during the day.

A reasonable mix 'n match of the meals in this section should typically result in approximately 1,600 calories consumed per day; this is in the mid-range for women and the low end of the program for men. Tweaking the daily calorie consumption upwards or downwards is as simple as adding or subtracting a little additional protein to your portions at lunch and dinner, choosing one salad dressing over the other, choosing lower or higher calorie veggies, or through choices of cooking options.

Just remember, Dynamic Dining Design is NOT about counting calories. Ultimately it is about:

- Reducing carbohydrate consumption to an acceptable minimal level;
- Eating healthy carbohydrates when you do consume them;
- Keeping your blood sugar fairly level throughout the day; and
- Eating the correct combinations of food in the correct proportions so your body resets and starts regulating your weight as it is supposed to.

The result will be that you will suddenly seem to develop your very own "magic genes" and your body will regulate your weight regardless of what you eat (as long as you stick to the program).

If you are following the Dynamic dining Design program and you have gotten down to or within range of your optimal weight, and you want to occasionally splurge, indulge yourself, or delight your palate, go ahead – don't feel guilty. As long as it is OCCASIONAL (meaning no more than once a month), it shouldn't affect your weight. But if every day becomes a splurge, you will soon be back at your old weight and your newly developed magic genes will abandon ship.

Keep your food journal for the first 3 or 4 months you are on the Dynamic Dining Design program. This is just until you get used to the portions and the program. After that, as long as you generally stick to the Carte Blanche foods and beverages, and you don't overdo Budgeted foods and beverages, you should be just fine without worrying about annoying details.

In the following charts the counts for calories, carbs, protein, fiber and sugar are ***GENERIC***. If you are eating food that is labeled, go by the information quoted on the label. If you are eating fresh, raw foods, the counts provided in the charts are perfectly adequate.

	Measure	Calories	Carbs *(g)*	Protein *(g)*	Fiber *(g)*	Sugar *(g)*
Breakfast #1						
Coffee – Fresh Brewed *(If instant, read label)*	1 cup (8 oz)	2	0	0	0	0
Artificial Sweetener	1 Packet	0	0	0	0	0
Half & Half *(read label)*	2 Tblspn	35	1	1	0	0
Eggs *(chicken)* *Poached or Boiled*	2 Lg Eggs	140	0	12.6	0	0
Total		**177**	**1**	**13.6**	**0**	**0**
Breakfast #2						
Tea – Freshly Brewed *(If instant, read label)*	1 cup (8 oz)	0	0	0	0	0
Artificial Sweetener	1 Packet	0	0	0	0	0
Half & Half *(read label)*	2 Tblspn	35	1	1	0	0
Eggs *(chicken)*	2 Lg Eggs	140	0	12.6	0	0
Scrambled or Fried w/ Allowed Oil	½ Tblspn	60	0	0	0	0
Total		**235**	**1**	**13.6**	**0**	**0**
Breakfast #3						
Coffee – Freshly Brewed *(If instant, read label)*	1 cup (8 oz)	2	0	0	0	0
Artificial Sweetener	1 Packet	0	0	0	0	0
Half & Half *(read label)*	2 Tblspn	35	1	1	0	0
Eggs *(chicken)* *Poached or Boiled*	2 Lg Eggs	140	0	12.6	0	0
English Muffin	½ Muffin	60	13	2	0.5	0
w/ Butter	½ Tblspn	50	0	0	0	0
Total		**287**	**14**	**15.6**	**0.5**	**0**

	Measure	Calories	Carbs (g)	Protein (g)	Fiber (g)	Sugar (g)
Basic Salad						
Lettuce *(any variety, incl mesclun greens)*	3-4 oz *(1 Lg Bowl)*	20	3.0	1.0	1.5	0
Tomato – Diced	¼ Cup	10	2.1	0	0.5	0
Cucumber – Diced	¼ Cup	4	0.7	0.2	0.3	0
Sprouts	2 Tblspn	3	0	0	0	0
Total		**37**	**5.8**	**1.2**	**2.3**	**0**
Dressing #1 – Oil & Vinegar						
Allowed Oil	1 Tblspn	120	0	0	0	0
Red Wine Vinegar	2 Tblspn	10	0	0	0	0
Herbs/Salt/Pepper	To Taste	1	0	0	0	0
Total		**131**	**0**	**0**	**0**	**0**
Dressing #2 – Bottled						
Spritz On Dressings *Wishbone Balsamic Breeze*	10 Spritzs	20	0	0	0	0
Total		**20**	**0**	**0**	**0**	**0**
Protein Salad ***(Examples)***						
Scoop any of following: *Tuna, Ham, Chicken, Turkey, Smoked Turkey, Crab, or Lobster **Salad***	6 oz. Scoop	180	4.0	21.0	2.0	1.0
OR						
Ham/Turkey/Cheese Pinwheels	6 oz	300	0	16.0	0	0
OR						
Sirloin Tips	6 oz	320	0	45.0	0	0
OR						
Grilled Chicken Strips	6 oz	240	0	32.0	0	0
OVER BASIC SALAD						

	Measure	Calories	Carbs (g)	Protein (g)	Fiber (g)	Sugar (g)
Lunch #1						
Tuna Salad	6 oz Scoop	180	4.0	21.0	2.0	1.0
OVER Basic Salad	Lg Bowl	37	5.8	1.4	2.5	0
Bok Choi – *Steamed OR*	1 Cup	20	3.0	2.5	2.8	>1.0
Sautéed w/ Butter	½ Tblspn	55	0	0	0	0
Total		**292**	**12.8**	**24.9**	**7.3**	**>2.0**
Lunch #2						
Basic Salad	Lg Bowl	37	5.8	1.4	2.5	0
Dressing #2	10 Spritzs	20	0	0	0	0
Chicken Breast – Grilled	6 oz	240	0	32.0	0	0
Green Beans – *Steamed*	1 Cup	35	8.0	2.5	4.0	1.0
OR Sautéed w/ Butter	½ Tblspn	55	0	0	0	0
Total		**387**	**13.8**	**35.9**	**6.5**	**1.0**
Lunch #3						
Basic Salad	Lg Bowl	37	5.8	1.4	2.5	0
Dressing #1	3 Tblspn	131	0	0	0	0
Hamburger Patty	6 oz	390	0	36.0	0	0
w/ Cheese	2 Slices	150	2.0	10.0	0	0
Mayonnaise	1 Tblspn	90	0	2.0	0	0
Mustard	1 Tblspn	5	0	0	0	0
Chopped Onion & Tomato	1 Cup	50	8.0	0	2.0	3.0
Total		**853**	**15.8**	**49.4**	**4.5**	**3.0**
Lunch #4						
Turkey/Cheese Rollups	6 oz	271	0	21.0	2.0	1.0
OVER Basic Salad	Lg Bowl	37	5.8	1.4	2.5	0
Bok Choi – *Steamed OR*	1 Cup	20	3.0	2.5	2.8	>1.0
Sautéed w/ Butter	½ Tblspn	55	0	0	0	0
Total		**383**	**8.8**	**24.9**	**7.3**	**>2.0**
Lunch #5						
Basic Salad	Lg Bowl	37	5.8	1.4	2.5	0
Dressing #2	10 Spritzs	20	0	0	0	0
Chicken Salad	6 oz	360	0	32.0	1.0	0
Green Beans *Almandine*	1 Cup	35	8.0	2.5	4.0	1.0
Total		**452**	**13.8**	**35.9**	**7.5**	**0**

	Measure	Calories	Carbs (g)	Protein (g)	Fiber (g)	Sugar (g)
Lunch #6						
Basic Salad	Lg Bowl	37	5.8	1.4	2.5	0
Dressing #2	10 Spritzs	20	0	0	0	0
Whole Shrimp – *Boiled*	6 oz	165	0	36.0	0	0
OR Sautéed w/ Butter	½ Tblspn	55	0	0	0	0
OR *w/ Remoulade Sauce (mayo/mustard/lemon juice)*	2 Tblspn	180	0	0	0	0
Asparagus – *Steam or grill*	1 Cup	40	7.4	4.0	4.0	1.0
Total		**497**	**13.2**	**41.4**	**6.5**	**1.0**
Lunch #7						
Basic Salad	Lg Bowl	37	5.8	1.4	2.5	0
Dressing #1	3 Tblspn	131	0	0	0	0
Veal – *Roast or grilled*	6 oz	330	0	54.0	0	0
Kale – Steamed	1 Cup	35	6.0	2.0	7.0	1.0
Total		**533**	**11.8**	**57.4**	**9.5**	**1.0**
Lunch #8						
Basic Salad	Lg Bowl	37	5.8	1.4	2.5	0
Dressing #2	10 Spritzs	20	0	0	0	0
Filet of Sole – *Broiled*	6 oz	204	0	42.0	0	0
OR *Sautéed w/ Butter*	1Tblspn	110	0	0	0	0
Fennel – *Roasted*	1 Cup	50	9.0	1.0	4.0	0
Total		**421**	**14.8**	**44.4**	**6.5**	**0**
Lunch #9						
Basic Salad	Lg Bowl	37	5.8	1.4	2.5	0
Dressing #2	10 Spritzs	20	0	0	0	0
Skirt Steak – *Broiled*	6 oz	450	0	48.0	0	0
Corn – *(On Cob or Kernels)*	1 Cup	120	16.0	6.0	6.0	6.0
Total		**627**	**21.8**	**55.4**	**8.5**	**6.0**
Lunch #10						
Basic Salad	Lg Bowl	37	5.8	1.4	2.5	0
Dressing #2	10 Spritzs	20	0	0	0	0
Crab Cocktail	6 oz	162	0	30.0	0	0
w/ Remoulade Sauce (mayo/mustard/lemon juice)	2 Tblspn	180	0	0	0	0
Asparagus – *Steam or grill*	1 Cup	40	7.4	4.0	4.0	1.0
Total		**452**	**13.8**	**35.9**	**7.5**	**0**

	Measure	Calories	Carbs (g)	Protein (g)	Fiber (g)	Sugar (g)
Dinner #1						
Basic Salad	Lg Bowl	37	5.8	1.4	2.5	0
Dressing #2	10 Spritzs	20	0	0	0	0
Tuna Steak – *Broiled*	8 oz	360	0	56.0	0	0
Celery – *Roasted*	¾ Cup	15	3.3	1.0	1.5	1.0
Broccoli – *Steamed*	¾ Cup	30	6.0	3.0	1.2	1.5
Total		**462**	**15.1**	**61.4**	**5.2**	**2.5**
Dinner #2						
Basic Salad	Lg Bowl	37	5.8	1.4	2.5	0
Dressing #2	10 Spritzs	20	0	0	0	0
Leg Lamb – *Roast or Broil*	8 oz	560	0	60.0	0	0
Kale – *Roasted*	1 Cup	35	6.0	2.0	7.0	>1.0
Celeriac – *Mashed*	¾ Cup	46	6.5	2.0	0	0
Total		**698**	**18.3**	**65.4**	**9.5**	**>1.0**
Dinner #3						
Basic Salad	Lg Bowl	37	5.8	1.4	2.5	0
Dressing #2	10 Spritzs	20	0	0	0	0
Chicken – *Roast or Broil*	8 oz	432	0	64.0	0	0
Green Beans – *Almandine*	1 Cup	35	8.0	2.5	4.0	1.0
Cabbage – *Boiled*	1 Cup	34	7.0	1.6	4.2	3.5
Total		**558**	**20.8**	**69.5**	**10.7**	**4.5**
Dinner #4						
Basic Salad	Lg Bowl	37	5.8	1.4	2.5	0
Dressing #2	10 Spritzs	20	0	0	0	0
Ostrich Medallion – ***Broil***	8 oz	368	0	48.0	0	0
Chard – ***Boiled or Steamed***	1 Cup	35	6.0	2.0	7.0	2.0
Celeriac – *Mashed*	¾ Cup	46	6.5	2.0	0	0
Total		**506**	**18.3**	**53.4**	**9.5**	**2.0**
Dinner #5						
Basic Salad	Lg Bowl	37	5.8	1.4	2.5	0
Dressing #2	10 Spritzs	20	0	0	0	0
Duck – *Roasted*	8 oz	760	0	40.0	0	0
Celery – *Roasted*	¾ Cup	15	3.3	1.0	1.5	1.0
Red Cabbage – ***Boiled***	¾ Cup	66	7.0	1.6	3.0	3.0
Total		**898**	**16.1**	**44.0**	**7.0**	**4.0**

	Measure	Calories	Carbs (g)	Protein (g)	Fiber (g)	Sugar (g)
Dinner #6						
Basic Salad	Lg Bowl	37	5.8	1.4	2.5	0
Dressing #2	10 Spritzs	20	0	0	0	0
Veal Chop – *Grilled*	8 oz	440	0	72.0	0	0
Asparagus – *Steam or Grill*	1 Cup	40	7.4	4.0	4.0	1.0
Potato – ***Baked or Roasted***	1 Small	100	26.0	4.0	3.0	2.0
Total		**637**	**39.2**	**81.4**	**9.5**	**2.0**
Dinner #7						
Seaweed Salad	1 Medium	85	4.0	2.0	5.0	0
Sashimi & Sushi – Fish	8 oz	320	0	52.0	0	0
Sticky Rice	¼ Cup	160	32.0	3.0	0	0
Bok Choi – ***Steamed***	1 Cup	20	3.0	2.5	2.8	>1.0
Total		**565**	**39.0**	**59.5**	**7.8**	**>1.0**
Dinner #8						
Basic Salad	Lg Bowl	37	5.8	1.4	2.5	0
Dressing #2	10 Spritzs	20	0	0	0	0
Flounder Filet – ***Baked***	8 oz	272	0	56.0	0	0
Brussel Sprouts – ***Roast***	1 Cup	60	12.0	2.0	7.0	1.0
Mustard Greens – ***Boiled***	1 Cup	35	6.0	2.0	7.0	0.0
Total		**424**	**23.8**	**61.4**	**16.5**	**1.0**
Dinner #9						
Basic Salad	Lg Bowl	37	5.8	1.4	2.5	0
Dressing #2	10 Spritzs	20	0	0	0	0
London Broil – ***Grill/Slice***	8 oz	400	0	48.0	0	0
Broccoli – ***Steamed***	1½ Cup	60	12.0	6.0	2.4	3.0
Total		**517**	**17.8**	**55.4**	**4.9**	**3.0**
Dinner #10						
Basic Salad	Lg Bowl	37	5.8	1.4	2.5	0
Dressing #1	3 Tblspns	131	0	0	0	0
Lobster – ***Steam or Broil***	8 oz	224	0	48.0	0	0
w/ Drawn Butter	1 Tblspn	110	0	0	0	0
Asparagus – *Steam or Grill*	1 Cup	40	7.4	4.0	4.0	1.0
Total		**542**	**13.2**	**53.4**	**6.5**	**1.0**

Appendix #6:
Your Daily Food Journal – Sample

	Measure	Calories	Carbs *(g)*	Protein *(g)*	Fiber *(g)*	Sugar *(g)*
Breakfast						
Sub-Total		0	0	0	0	0
Snack #1						
Sub-Total		0	0	0	0	0
Lunch						
Sub-Total		0	0	0	0	0
Snack #2						
Sub-Total		0	0	0	0	0
Dinner						
Sub-Total		0	0	0	0	0
Total For Day		0	0	0	0	0

References

CDC Statistics on U.S. Overweight/Obesity 2013-2014.

World Health Organization on Global Obesity 2014.

Hypnosis for Weight Control, 2010, Mayo Clinic.

Diabetes Trends 1990-1998, Diabetes Care Magazine, September 2000 Issue.

Cholesterol in the Diet: The Long Slide from Public Menace to No "Appreciable" Effect, Washington Post, Feb. 19, 2015; By Peter Whoriskey .

Eggs Are Okay Again, Washington Post, Jan 7, 2016, By Ariana Eunjung Cha.

Use of Cholesterol-lowering Medications in the United States from 1991 to 1997, David Siegel, MD, MPH, Julio Lopez, PharmD, Joy Meier, PharmD.

Diabetes, Cholesterol, BP: Normal is no longer normal, by Dr. Zoe Harcombe, PH.D.

Thyroid Screening Neglected in Hypercholesterolemia, May 2, 2013, Medscape.

American Association of Clinical Endocrinologists

Many Obese Americans Struggle With Stigma, Discrimination, Poll Finds, US News and World Reports, August 23, 2012, By Amanda Gardner.

Study Concludes 'Fat-ism' Is More Widespread Than Racism, Huffington Post, April 10, 2008.

Stigma Against Fat People the Last Acceptable Prejudice, Studies Find, ABC News, Jan. 22, 2013 .

What's Fair? Equity in Educational Practice, Educational Horizons, 2005, VOL 84; 1, By Gary K. Clabaugh and Alison A. Clabaugh.

Controversy: Is It Fair for Ob-gyns to Turn Away Patients for Being Fat?, Glamour Magazine, August 2011, Health, By Ginny Graves.

Doctors Back Denial of Treatment for Smokers and the Obese, The Guardian, April 28, 2012.

Browsers Book of Beginnings, by Charles Panati.

Hominoid Origins, Nature Education Knowledge 6(7):4, (2015), By MacLatchy, L. M., Sanders, W. J. & Wuthrich, C. L.

Human Evolution Timeline, Smithsonian Museum of Natural History website: humanorigins.si.edu, March 9, 2017.

The clinical consequences of obstructive sleep apnea and associated excessive sleepiness. J. Fam Pract., Aug. 2008, By M. Hirshkowitz.

Diagnosis and Treatment of Obstructive Sleep Apnea in Adulta, Bloomington (MN): Institute for Clinical Systems Improvement (ICSI); Mar. 2007.

Association Between Obstructive Sleep Apnea and Weight Gain Found, American Academy of Sleep Medicine, (2009).

Sleep, Sleep Disorders, and Biological Rhythms, The National Institute of Health.

Obesity and sleep, National Sleep Foundation, (2009).

Light at Night Increases Body Mass by Shifting the Time of Food Intake, Proceedings of the National Academy of Sciences, (2010), by L. K. Fonken, J. W. Workman, J. C. Walton, Z. M. Weil, J. S. Morris, A. Haim, & R. J. Nelson

Melatonin: Hormone of Sleep and Much More, By Earl Mindell, R.Ph., Ph.D. and Melissa Block

Cancer Causes Control, Nighttime Light Level Co-distributes with Breast Cancer Incidence Worldwide, 21:2059-2068, DOI 10.1007/s10552-010-9624-4, 2010, by I. Kloog, R. G. Stevens, A. Haim, B. A. Portnov.

Night-Shift Work Linked to Cancer, USA Today, Nov 29, 2007 By H. Darr Beiser.

Watch Out: Daylight Saving Time May Cause Heart Attack Spike, Live Science, 2015, By Laura Geggel

Thyroid Hormone Disorders. May 2001, By Jennifer A. Phillips

Nutrition and Physical Degeneration, By Weston Price

Lick the Sugar Habit, By Nancy Appleton, Ph.D

Little Sugar Addicts, By Kathleen DesMaisons, Ph.D.

Food Irradiation, Academic Press, 1986, By Walter M. Urbain.

High-Dose Irradiation: (Wholesomeness of Food irradiated with Doses Above 10kGy), Joint FAO/IAEA/WHO Study Group, Geneva, Switzerland, 1997.

Food Irradiation – the problems and concerns, Position Paper of The US Food Commission, July 2002

Dangers of Pasteurization and Homogenization, (Nov. 2010) Prevent Disease.com

Mercury and Tuna: U.S. Advice Leaves Lots of Questions, Wall Street Journal, August 1, 2005, By Peter Waldman, Staff Reporter

FDA issues a nationwide recall of all over-the-counter dietary supplements containing 100 milligrams or more of L-*Tryptophan. By 1990 the Centers for Disease Control and Prevention confirm over 1,500 cases of EMS, including 38 deaths, and FDA prohibits the importation of l-tryptophan*, Significant Dates in U.S. Food and Drug Law History, FDA, 1989. Source: FDA Website.

Prozac A Breakthrough Drug for Depression, Newsweek VOLUME CXV, NO. 13, March 26, 1990

The FDA Ban of L-Tryptophan: Politics, Profits and Prozac , "Social Policy", Vol. 26, No. 2 Winter 1995, By Dean Wolfe Manders, Ph.D.

Johnson and Johnson's Recall of Children's Tylenol and Other Children's Medicines, Statement of Joshua M. Sharfstein, M.D., Principal Deputy Commissioner, U.S. Food and Drug Administration, Congressional Testimony, Sept. 30, 2010

A Brief History of the [1982] Tylenol Poisonings, Time Magazine, Feb. 9, 2009, By Dan Fletcher

Recalls are making antacids harder to find, USA Today Mar 6, 2011, By Dana Hunsinger Benbow

Lipitor (atorvastatin) 40 mg: Recall Specific Bottles, FDA Safety Alerts, Dec. 23, 2010

Perrier Recalls Its Water in U.S. After Benzene Is Found in Bottles, NY Times, Feb. 10, 1990, By George James

List of Toothpaste Brands Contaminated with Antifreeze Chemical, NBC News, June 1, 2007

How Do Health Plans Pay Physicians?, University of Minnesota, Health Plan Task Force. By Matthew L. Maciejewski.

Financial Incentives, How Does Your Doctor Get Paid? PBS Frontline, By Mark Hagland

How Medical Care is Being Corrupted, NY Times, Nov 18, 2014, By Pamela Hartzband and Jerome Groopman

JOSEPH MAIO; JO ANN MAIO; and GARY BENDER, ON BEHALF OF THEMSELVES AND ALL OTHERS SIMILARLY SITUATED **v.** AETNA INC.; AETNA-US HEALTHCARE, INC;

AETNA-U.S. HEALTHCARE OF ARIZONA INC.; AETNA-U.S. HEALTHCARE OF CALIFORNIA INC.; AETNA-U.S. HEALTHCARE INC. (COLORADO); AETNA HEALTH PLANS OF SOUTHERN NEW ENGLAND, INC.; AETNA-U.S. HEALTHCARE, INC. (DELAWARE); AETNA-U.S. HEALTHCARE INC. (FLORIDA); AETNA-U.S. HEALTHCARE OF GEORGIA INC.; AETNA-U.S. HEALTHCARE OF ILLINOIS; AETNA-U.S. HEALTHCARE INC. (KENTUCKY); AETNA-U.S. HEALTHCARE INC. (LOUISIANA); AETNA-U.S. HEALTHCARE INC. (MASSACHUSETTS); AETNA-U.S. HEALTHCARE INC. (MICHIGAN); AETNA-HEALTH PLANS OF NEW JERSEY, INC.; AETNA-U.S. HEALTHCARE INC. (NEW YORK); AETNA-U.S. HEALTHCARE OF THE CAROLINAS; AETNA-U.S. HEALTHCARE INC. (OHIO); AETNA-U.S. HEALTHCARE INC. (PENNSYLVANIA); AETNA HEALTH PLANS OF CENTRAL AND EASTERN PENNSYLVANIA, INC.; AETNA HEALTH PLANS OF WESTERN PENNSYLVANIA, INC; AETNA HEALTH PLANS OF TENNESSEE, INC.; AETNA-U.S. HEALTHCARE INC. (TEXAS); AETNA-U.S. HEALTHCARE OF NORTH TEXAS INC.; AETNA-U.S. HEALTHCARE INC. (VIRGINIA); AETNA-U.S. HEALTHCARE OF WASHINGTON INC. JOSEPH MAIO; JO ANN MAIO; GARY BENDER, **Appellants; 221 F.3d 472 (3rd Cir. 2000), No. 99-1854.**

More Employees Covered by Self-Insured Health Plans, CEBS, 2012, By Stephen Miller.

Health Care Costs and Quality, (2008), By Stan Lass.

Ethics Pinched by the System, USA Today, By David Leon Moore.

Physicians Hands Are Tied When it Comes to Negotiating for YOU or for Themselves, Ethical Health Partnerships, 2004, By Dawn Lipthrott.

CDC BMI Calculator:
https://www.cdc.gov/healthyweight/assessing/bmi/adult_BMI/english_bmi_calculator/bmi_calculator.html

Index

I

J

K

L

M

V

W

For more information
and weight loss support,
please visit our website:

www.The3dDiet.com

ABOUT THE AUTHOR

Victoria Rosenthal's lifelong struggle with her weight in many ways shaped her life. The myriad facts she has discovered over decades of research about weight and weight loss have culminated in this book. Strong willed and persistent, Victoria successfully educated herself about weight loss and the medical facts no one wants us to know despite the numerous barriers purposely erected by the medical industry, the pharmaceutical industry, the insurance industry, the food industry, and the government, as well as the enormous amount of mis-information promulgated by all of them.

Writing from the trenches of her own experience, Victoria shares the straight skinny about weight and how to lose it – facts that no one else will tell you!

Currently residing with her beloved husband and their adorable cats, Victoria has had many careers throughout her journey and considers herself to be something of a jack-of-all-trades. A happy workaholic who travels extensively, by train, plane, and her own imagination, Victoria considers her husband, their cats, and the workaholism to be fairly permanent; everything else is a moveable feast.

Made in the USA
Monee, IL
08 November 2026

67379942R00173